The Middle Way Diet
for Health and Fitness

The Middle Way Diet for Health and Fitness

Healthy Mind and Body

Emil Payman Moshedi, M.D.

iUniverse, Inc.
New York Lincoln Shanghai

The Middle Way Diet for Health and Fitness
Healthy Mind and Body

Copyright © 2007 by Emil Payman Moshedi

All rights reserved. No part of this book may be used or reproduced by any means, graphic, electronic, or mechanical, including photocopying, recording, taping or by any information storage retrieval system without the written permission of the publisher except in the case of brief quotations embodied in critical articles and reviews.

iUniverse books may be ordered through booksellers or by contacting:

iUniverse
2021 Pine Lake Road, Suite 100
Lincoln, NE 68512
www.iuniverse.com
1-800-Authors (1-800-288-4677)

Because of the dynamic nature of the Internet, any Web addresses or links contained in this book may have changed since publication and may no longer be valid.

You should not undertake any diet/exercise regimen recommended in this book before consulting your physician.

Neither the author nor the publisher shall be responsible or liable for any loss or damage allegedly arising as a consequence of your use or application of any information or suggestions contained in this book.

ISBN: 978-0-595-41097-2 (pbk)
ISBN: 978-0-595-85456-1 (ebk)

Printed in the United States of America

Contents

Chapter 1 Health is Your Choice 1
    Healthy Today is Pleasure Today 1
    Stop Need To Gain Satisfaction 3
    Become Healthy or Accept Obesity 4
    Decide to Learn How to Be Fit 4
    Choose Health or Accept Consequences 5

Chapter 2 Think Your Way to a Healthy Body 7
    Healthy Body and Mind 7
    Physical Domino Effect 8
    You Are What You Choose to Eat 9
    Taking Care of Your Mind 10
    Learning the Middle Way 11
    Understanding Your Desires 13

Chapter 3 Your Middle Way 14
    Map Your Way to Health 14
    Examine Yourself to Find Your Way 15

Chapter 4 Metabolism and Weight 18
    The Reality of Weight 18
    The Weight Formula 20
    The Weight Formula in Depth 21

Chapter 5 The Mind Diet 24
    Healthy Food Tastes Good 25
    Are you Hungry When You Eat 26

Eating Healthy Is Happy 27
Eating Less is More Pleasurable 28
Culture and Perspective on Fat and Fit 29
Hunger in Your Stomach Not Your Brain 29
Strengthen Your Awareness 30

Chapter 6 The Practical Diet 33
Practical Diet Ideas 35
Fat Deposition Control 38
Understand and Accept Hunger 39
More Tips 42

Chapter 7 The Ratio Diet 43
Proteins 43
Fiber 45
Carbohydrates 46
Fats 48
Water 49
Basic Meal Selection 49
Label Criteria 51

Chapter 8 Exercise in the Middle Way 53
The Scale is Your Report Card 54
Exercise Improves Your Quality of Life 55
Make it a Priority in Your Schedule 56
Learn to Make Exercise Part of Your Life 56

Chapter 9 Guideposts for Healthy Living 63

References 69
About the Author 71

Chapter 1

Health is Your Choice

Healthy Today is Pleasure Today

Living a healthy and happy life is a choice. You can reduce your chances of serious disease if you choose a healthy way of living. Many diseases, such as common colds, flu, hypertension, high cholesterol, diabetes, heart disease, stroke, and many cancers, can be directly attributed to the choices you make. The numbers of people who suffer from these diseases could be significantly reduced if more people lived healthier lives.

Disease is a natural part of being human and cannot be completely eliminated. However, some people get sick and die early because of poor choices they have made. One of the most deadly lifestyle choices we make involves our weight. Eliminate obesity, and the incidence of the most common causes of death would be significantly reduced.

Many people seem to think that living a healthy life means that they have to stop enjoying their lives. But this isn't true. Being healthy will enhance the quality of your life. As you learn the truth about being healthy, your perspective will change. Living healthy will make today and tomorrow better, and will help you be happier if you do happen to live to 100.

But the goal of this book is not necessarily to help you live to 100. Becoming physically fit will increase your chances of a longer life, but it will not guarantee it. Even physically fit people get sick and die young. I recommend that you follow my motto:

> Prepare to live for tomorrow, but be ready to live forever;
> prepare to live forever, but be ready to die tomorrow.

Whether you live another 100 days or 100 years is not as important as living well today. Living healthy today can improve the quality of your life as soon as tomorrow. If you live healthy now, you'll also be better prepared to enjoy life when you are older. There are many other benefits. Living healthy can:

- relieve your ailments and therefore increase the quality of your life
- significantly improve your emotional and mental health, elevating your mood and your pleasure in living
- supply you with a more fit and functional body
- leave your body capable in old age without pain
- strengthen your immunity so that you are less likely to have minor illnesses
- decrease your chances of getting debilitating or life ending disease

The Middle Way Diet offers you a realistic way to attain a healthy mind and body. The Middle Way Diet is based on a philosophy that recognizes extremism in ourselves and the world, but advises us to find and stay on the metaphorical middle road. This diet takes a balanced approach to health and fitness. It avoids extreme ideas, views, and practices. Remember that the power to achieve health and fitness belongs to you. No outside force, being, individual, pill, or potion—not even this book—will give you that power. The power is yours. The Middle Way Diet reminds you to see and believe for yourself. It may be hard for you to see the truth, because your perspective on food and exercise has been shaped by false, extremist ideas. Our families, communities, culture, and the media have taught us that we have to overindulge our senses to find happiness in life. This false idea has hidden what you already know deep down inside. You already know what it takes to be healthy and fit. You already know that you need a balanced lifestyle similar to the middle way approach. You know that both overindulgence and deprivation are unhealthy. To follow the Middle Way Diet, listen to that voice inside you that already knows what to do.

Stop Need To Gain Satisfaction

Think about the things you think you need. You decide what you think you need. When you constantly need things, you create dissatisfaction and unhappiness in your life. I'm not referring to food or water or to basic needs that need to be met, but to those "needs" that are really "wants": the constant craving for bigger and better things. If you are unable to get what you want, you become unhappy with unfulfilled desire. Even if you get what you thought you needed, you get only a brief sense of satisfaction. When your satisfaction passes, you are left dissatisfied, longing for the next "fix" to satisfy yourself. The initial feeling of satisfaction passes because you cannot stop time. You cannot take a picture of the feeling and savor it forever.

I hope you'll begin to realize that this cycle of temporary satisfaction followed by dissatisfaction arises when you believe that you need things. Don't believe what you've been told by advertisements and by others about what you need. Decide for yourself what you need and why you need it. As simple as deciding to move a finger you can consciously manipulate your desires. Become aware of your mind's desires. See them for what they are. Consciously step back and monitor what your mind is craving. By practicing, you can learn to have conscious awareness of your emotions and desires.

Learning to decide for yourself happens gradually, not overnight. Over time, you can become aware of your desires and your actions. Then you can make yourself happy and content without depending on unreasonable desires.

Please remember that how you feel about yourself should have little to do with your physical appearance. Start to let go of your attachment to your physical appearance. Wanting to be beautiful is just another desire, achieved or not, that never leads to long lasting happiness and fulfillment. Your true happiness comes from within yourself. Fat or thin, ultimately your happiness is a state of mind. Happiness resides within your brain, and should have little to do with how you look—but it should not be at the expense of being physically unfit and unhealthy.

I understand that you might want to start a diet and fitness program for aesthetic reasons. I also strongly recommend that you start to accept yourself for who you are. You need to lose your desire to be thin just so you can conform to others' expectations. If you are too strongly motivated by that desire, you will risk unhealthy obsessions and weight-loss extremes. You may cause yourself physical harm because your body and mind are not in balance.

Become Healthy or Accept Obesity

You must first decide if you are fat. If you are fat, you have to accept the reality of your situation. Then you have to decide if you really want to be fit. It is your decision to make. There is nothing wrong or shameful about being fat and happy if in fact you are happy. You could continue to live the way you are as long as you are willing to accept the negative health consequences. You do not have to accept societal pressure to be fit if that is not what you want. Either accept it emotionally and stop dwelling on it or do something about.

If you have decided to do something about it, consider if the mental anguish of always wanting to be fit is easier for you to accept than the work of actually losing the weight. You have to decide if it means that much to you to live a longer functional life. Motivate yourself by realizing that if you don't lose the weight you will suffer numerous negative health effects. Motivate yourself by deciding that you don't want to accept becoming less functional and dying sooner because of obesity. Many people will simply avoid the reality of their situation until it is too late. Think about it now and make a lasting decision and commitment. At first, these statements seem obvious to you. But have you taken the time to really comprehend the ramifications? These statements are also blunt, and may be hard for you to hear. It is important to think about this over and over until you truly understand and see the reality of your situation.

Many people avoid the reality of their situation until it is too late. They try to convince themselves to accept the consequences of being fat. They usually change their perspective after the first heart attack. Please decide now before it is too late. You may not get a second chance.

Decide to Learn How to Be Fit

All of us have a certain amount of difficulty learning new information and skills. Learning how to live healthy is no different. If you are determined and persistent, you'll learn and know how to live this positive way. As with everything you need to learn, your success depends on your motivation. If you sincerely want to live healthy, you can learn how.

The reason there are so many diet plans and scams is that people want to buy a way to be thin. Yet such a way has not yet been bottled or published. Everyone wants the easy way, but there is no easy way—except to learn and practice. You have to achieve weight loss on your own.

Living healthy may not be easy at first, but it can become easier and more natural with practice. Learning new things is always difficult at first. It is no different than learning to play an instrument, play a sport, learn a new job, etc. When we learn new things it sometimes seems overwhelming and impossibly difficult. Eventually with persistence we learn. Ultimately, it becomes so easy that we wonder what the big deal was in the first place.

Are you ready to do something about changing your way of life? You have to have the right reasons. You have to really be motivated. Anyone can do it, but most people don't because they don't make the effort required. If being fit were easy, everyone would be.

So your next step is to decide, deep down, that being fit is what you want. Accept the personal responsibility for your own success or failure. If you don't really want to do what is required, stop! Stop the irrationality of repeated attempts that are doomed to failure. Why make half-hearted attempts, hoping this time you'll lose weight? Failing over and over just adds more dissatisfaction to your life. Decide that *this time, you will succeed!*

Choose Health or Accept Consequences

Once and for all, decide you're not happy as you are now. Decide that you want to change. Know in your mind that you can and will make it happen. Start to believe that your mind has the power to make it happen. All the things that you have done and achieved started in your mind. This will be no different. Your mind is powerful and can do many amazing things. Just as your mind turns these pages, it also creates your emotions and desires. Your mind decides what and how much to eat. It decides to exercise. The outcome is your mind's responsibility. Accept success or failure without blaming outside forces.

If you choose to be unbalanced you should also be prepared to accept the consequences. Unhealthy habits increase the risk of developing irreversible disease. There are always examples or anecdotes of individuals with unhealthy habits that are lucky enough to live long lives. Are those risks that you are willing to take? If you take those risks, be prepared to deal with the possible consequences. Smokers are at higher risk of developing emphysema and some will have to live attached to an oxygen tank. Alcoholics risk liver failure. The obese are highly prone to diabetes and high blood pressure leading to heart attacks and strokes. Consciously decide in advance that you knowingly accept the consequences of your lifestyle. If you accept that your life of so-called pleasure and excess is the way you want to live and die that is fine. Realize however that many of these same people often change their perspective with the onset of irreversible illness. They no longer say that smoking, drinking, and excess eating is what makes life pleasurable. They can now envision a life without the poor habits. If fact, they will crave a second chance.

Furthermore, many mildly obese people are highly critical and even disgusted by severely obese people. You have probably seen the image of an obese person confined to his bed and thought, *How pathetic to be out of control.* Don't judge others; rather, examine yourself. Just as you see the weakness in others you have to see the weakness in yourself. You may be mildly obese, but realize that a fit person may see you just as grotesquely as you view people that are fatter than you.

But start to judge yourself. We all have our problems and lack conscious awareness in different ways. Excessive eating is not much different than other bad habits such as smoking, drinking, and drug use. You need to adjust your perspective. No one is perfect. Realize that you harbor these critical, perhaps accurate, thoughts of others. However, you really should be looking inward to yourself.

Pleasure in life is derived in the process of living a healthy, balanced lifestyle. Pleasures in life are not what you have come to believe they are. Re-examine your priorities and what truly brings you long-lasting and deep satisfaction. Then you will realize that excesses and overindulgence are not satisfying. You might ask, what is the pleasure in life without eating as much as you desire. Imagine, then, how you would answer an alcoholic who asked what the pleasure in life would be without beer and wine.

As you accept your mind's role in this change, I ask you to respect your body, too. Be aware of your body's needs. Let your body know you want to take care of it. Make a resolution to change any body-harming habits—smoking, excessive drinking, drug use, excessive eating—because having a healthy body helps make your life pleasurable. When you take care of your body, you can envision a life without poor habits. And you will be the one who reaps the benefits.

Much of the pleasure in life is derived from living in a healthy, balanced way. Think about the activities that bring you long-lasting, deep satisfaction. I hope you conclude that excesses and overindulgence are not satisfying. And I hope you will begin to accept the goal of choosing health for yourself. With that goal before you, you can next begin to gain a healthy body and a healthy mind, which I'll explain in the next chapter.

Chapter 2

Think Your Way to a Healthy Body

Healthy Body and Mind

The Middle Way Diet can lead you toward gaining a healthy body and a healthy mind. Following this path to health and happiness requires awareness of all aspects of life.

A healthy body supports a healthy mind. In turn, a healthy mind supports a healthy body. When your mind is in a healthy state of consciousness, you can more easily maintain your body in a healthy state of being. Similarly, when your body is healthy, it will help keep your mind healthy. When you are in a healthy state of mind, you realize that desire for dissatisfying things wastes your energy. Even when you have satisfied a desire, the sensation is often fleeting. After it passes, you'll have the same uneasy feeling of wanting—unless you make a conscious decision to stop the cycle.

Your healthy mind can think more clearly, guiding you to eat right and to exercise. Your body will become healthy and feel good. When your body is healthy, your heart will be strong as it pumps blood through open, unclogged arteries. Your brain will be nourished with good, healthy blood that stimulates a healthy happy mind. Together, the mind and the body create a healthy cycle and support one other.

Consider this: healthy feet allow you to jog, creating a healthy heart. A healthy heart allows good blood flow to the brain, creating healthy brain cells. Healthy brain cells create a healthy-thinking mind, which can consciously decide to go jogging. Thus, a healthy cycle is formed, and the process repeats and maintains itself.

On the other hand, an unhealthy mindset can lead to physical decline. Stress, for example, can suppress the immune system and make the body more susceptible to illness and disease. In turn, physical ailments can challenge the mind's ability to maintain happiness. Mental stress can harm the body, and physical illness can stress the mind. I'd like you also to understand the importance of the middle way approach. If jogging turns into excessive exercise, you may injure your knees, and your body and mind will suffer. If you don't exercise at all, your knees may last forever, but high blood pressure and cholesterol may ensure that the rest of your body does not last. If you exercise in excess, your heart may be ready for a marathon, but your knees won't be able to walk it. The middle way approach dictates that you need to find the right and reasonable balance to maintain a healthy cycle of mind and body health.

Physical Domino Effect

An example can show you the interrelationship of your body parts. Suppose you're sitting down to a meal. Here's what your body is going to do for you without your even thinking about it:

- Your healthy teeth allow you to chew food into the appropriate size for your stomach to digest.
- Your healthy stomach digests the food into the appropriate size for the small intestine.
- Your healthy small intestine extracts the carbohydrates to fuel your body.
- Your healthy small intestine also extracts the proteins and fats to maintain your body's structure.
- And your healthy small intestine extracts the minerals and vitamins to support your body's functions.
- Your healthy large intestine eliminates the unhealthy by-products from your food.

What an amazing system, right? But if any part of your body's system doesn't work appropriately, the other parts will be negatively affected. If your teeth don't function well, the stomach cannot effectively digest the largest piece of food. Also, if your small intestine can't extract the nutrients, your teeth will further degenerate. Without enough calcium, your bones will grow weaker, leading to such afflictions as osteoporosis, spinal degeneration, and hunchback. And these negative effects are just the beginning of a long list of possible results.

Such physical maladies that occur when the digestive system is out of balance can also affect the mind. For example, it is hard to find mental satisfaction from taking a walk after lunch if a poorly functioning digestive system has produced constipation and, over time, degenerative spinal pain. As another example, a person who is obese and has developed high blood pressure can suffer an eye stroke—a retinal occlusion—and lose vision. Not being able to see would cause stress to the mind.

I offer these examples to underline one fact: People who live in an unhealthy way can have less pleasure in their lives. If you have been living an unhealthy life, I hope you will rethink your approach and will make up your mind to live according to the healthy middle way. This will ultimately give you more pleasure and satisfaction.

You Are What You Choose to Eat

Your physical body is a biological machine made up of carbon atoms. These various atoms make up molecules, which in turn make up tissue, which makes up organs. The human body is not simply put together and maintained by replacing parts when they fail. The body is alive and is continuously being put together and taken apart as you eat and digest your food. Your body is in continuous development, maintenance, disintegration, and elimination.

For example, your bones are alive and in continuous flux and change. Within the bones are special cells called osteoblasts (pronounced AHS-tee-uh-blasts) that lay down new bone, and cells called osteoclasts (pronounced AHS-tee-uh-clasts) that reabsorb old bone. Both these types of cells are continuously working, taking away old bone and creating new bone to keep you strong. When you break a bone, the osteoblasts lay down new bone to fill in the gap in the break. At the same time, the osteoclasts remold the edges. The bone is continuously being put together and taken apart, continuously remodeling itself to be well and strong.

Just like bone, all the organs in your body are in continuous, living flux, growing and repairing themselves. Even your skin is regenerating while you are reading this chapter. Did you know that, each thirty days, your skin completely replaces itself? Every inch of your skin becomes brand new once a month!

A science fiction movie might show a high-tech creature that can repair a knife wound in a very short time—say, five seconds. But your body is high tech, too, and takes only a few weeks to heal even a badly cut finger—a *real* cut finger, not one invented for a science fiction film!

To grow and repair itself, your body uses a community of its parts, all working together interdependently to gather the necessary building blocks.

- Your lungs bring oxygen.
- Your digestive system brings amino acids that make proteins.
- Your digestive system also brings fatty acids that make up parts of the cells.
- Your blood delivers these building blocks by the pumping action of your heart through your arteries.
- Your kidneys and liver process and eliminate the waste byproducts.

If you eat a balanced, healthy diet, you give your body the materials it needs to function, grow, and repair itself properly. If you don't eat a balanced, healthy diet, your body cannot function or repair itself and eventually may fail. The saying you've heard many times—that you are what you eat—is very true. I prefer to say that you are what you *choose* to eat, because it is a choice. To live in a healthy way, you have to give your body the material it needs to work properly. You cannot deprive your body of the building blocks or poison it with unhealthy air, drink, and food, because then your body cannot function optimally.

Taking Care of Your Mind

I hope you are gradually realizing that your body has specific needs so that you can begin making conscious choices about what fuel to put into your body and how to treat it. The relationship between your body and your mind is critical in healthy living. Your mind helps you decide what to take into your body—that is, what to eat and drink. If you make uninformed choices without being aware of what your body requires, you and your body will suffer the consequences.

Your desires are created in your physical brain, and your mind controls your brain. Your mind tells your brain to do easy tasks like lifting your finger to turn a page or pulling up the corners of your mouth to smile at a friend. Your mind can also tell your brain to be happy and content without relying on unsatisfying, unhealthful foods or objects. An illustration of the interdependence of the parts of your mind would be that when a person takes part in loving relationships, that person will feel content and satisfied. If this same content, satisfied person is studying for school, his mind can more easily focus and learn. If he is competing in sports while content and satisfied, he will be more mentally prepared and can concentrate effectively. He may not be a first-place winner, but he is more likely to enjoy what he is doing.

On the other hand, a person who is not able to cope with stress at work may not be able to show love to his/her spouse and children. Without the mental health derived from giving and getting love from his family, he will find that his mind may be less able to handle the challenges at work. He may be so stressed that he will forget to eat correctly. He may skip a healthy lunch for a quick, unhealthy meal and afterward experience poor digestion and physical discomfort.

Learning the Middle Way

While many people tend toward an extreme—either eating too much or too little, exercising too much or not at all—you can develop a middle way approach. When your mind is aware and vigilant, you can maintain a healthy, balanced approach. Just as an athlete can learn to succeed physically by repetition and practice, you can develop your mental functioning.

A simple illustration is learning and memorizing. When you study in school, you are exercising your mind. Training your mind to learn a list of spelling words takes repetition and practice. The mind can also be trained to control emotions. You have probably achieved this type of learning already simply in the process of growing up into a mature adult.

When you were a child, you may have thrown a tantrum when you did not get what you wanted. Now that you're older, you don't have those tantrums. Through practice, training, and time, you matured and realized that tantrums were not an effective way to get what you wanted. Your adult mind has developed and matured. Keep in mind that you have trained your mind before, and you can do it again.

If we examine ourselves honestly, we can find immaturity within ourselves. The majority of us haven't fully grown up mentally. But we can try to become more mature through intentional awareness. When you are strongly inclined to avoid exercise or to eat more than you know is good for you, you can stop and think again. If you don't stuff yourself at a buffet breakfast, you will still have enough to eat, and you will have shown your mental maturity.

The reason you may not see your mental and emotional immaturity is that you don't think about it. Like most people, you believe that, since you're an adult, you have the answers and can control yourself. If you're driving and another driver cuts you off, you may reflexively get angry. You think your anger is appropriate because you rationalize that you have been wronged by the person who cut you off.

When the long line to check out at the grocery store irritates you, you may start grumbling. Your blood pressure and heart rate rise, and your healthy state of mind and body is disrupted. You may think this anger is the fault of someone else. Yet when you consider the situation with mental and emotional maturity, you may see that your reflexive response of irritation is an immature, illogical reaction.

Your irritation and anger are created by your mind. The situations I have described as examples did not infect your brain and cause your reaction. Your mind reacted reflexively, without awareness. You decided to get angry, just as easily as you decided what items to choose at the grocery store.

Instead of letting reflexive thought control you, you can choose to respond in a mature way. What does such a mature response involve?

- You can decide that the situation will pass and will soon be forgotten.
- You can realize that no long-term negative effects will result unless you let emotion govern your mind.

If your child had been standing in the line with you at the grocery store and started getting frustrated by the delay, you would probably take the opportunity to teach your child to relax. Now you can tell yourself that same message. The anger isn't in the air, and you didn't breathe it into your system. You create the emotion in your mind, and you can just as easily not create it. As anger arises, you can let it pass without allowing it to overwhelm you. Responding in this mature, rational way may take mental practice, and you can do it. Emotional and mental maturity helps you achieve peace and happiness within yourself.

Factors outside your control can influence your immature emotions. If you allow other influences to control you, you are likely to lose your conscious awareness and get carried away with emotion. Stress and anger, in response to the environment around you, only harm you by raising your pulse and blood pressure. Not only did your immature anger affect your own health, but now you are also affecting the peace and tranquility of your community. Many of the decisions you make can affect the health of the people around you—both positively and negatively. You already know this middle way approach. The fact that you would teach your child and not yourself illustrates that fact. The disconnect can be overcome by maintaining conscious awareness about your own ideas, thoughts, and behaviors as being separate from the world around you.

Understanding Your Desires

As a human, you desire things, including food, to secure a good feeling for yourself. But everything you take is borrowed, changed, and deposited. As you mature, you will understand that nothing lasts. It always changes.

For instance, you can desire to eat a delicious meal. You enjoy the anticipation of the food, and while you chew, the taste is fabulous. Unfortunately, you can't savor the taste over and over. By the time the food has reached your stomach, it becomes a completely different substance. It has changed entirely. What you anticipated and consumed as a delicious meal is transformed into nutrition—perhaps excess nutrition—and eventually is deposited back into the environment.

What you think about food depends upon how you view it. Your perspective of food on a plate is not the same as when that food is in your stomach, being digested, or when it is waiting in your body to be excreted as waste. The point is that you crave a food item as though it has a permanent effect on you. You falsely believe that when you eat it you will be happy. But your sense of fulfillment and happiness is temporary and does not last.

You can learn that what you crave to eat or achieve or acquire is never permanent. Eating meals, buying cars, and gaining promotions in business never secures a constant state of satisfaction for you. The pleasure of a meal is similar to the pleasure of hearing a funny joke that makes you laugh deep down inside. You know at that moment that this joke is hilarious, perhaps the funniest you ever heard. Unfortunately, you can't hold that moment forever. You can't even replicate it. Even if you listen to the joke over and over, you will never recreate that moment. What you thought was the funniest joke you ever heard, if told again and again, loses its humor and ability to bring you pleasure. You cannot save it. Enjoy it while the pleasure lasts because you can't put it in your pocket or in the bank. Your emotional attachment to food is the same way.

In the next chapter, I show you how to develop your personal map for living in the present and enjoying everything—including food and exercise—in the moment.

Chapter 3

Your Middle Way

Map Your Way to Health

A map is a directional guide telling you how to get somewhere. This book can become your map that shows you how to get where you want to be with respect to diet and fitness. This book offers you a map, a framework on how to live well. Without a guide you can become lost and confused.

But the personal map of this book is only your starting point, not the final answer. You can think rationally and consciously as you decide for yourself what to do and what to choose. You can learn to analyze the world critically, asking questions and expecting answers that make sense. Don't take an explanation as fact just because it is written in this or any book. After you read this book, you may be sold on the methodology explained here, but strong emotional feelings do not make changes come into fruition. You can develop a system that truly makes rational sense for you. Only believing won't make anything happen for you.

Believing a fact or statement involves trust, and trust is built on experiences. Having belief is important, but finding out that what you believe is actually true by experiencing it will be much more powerful for you.

When you refer to a map, you generally believe that the map is accurate, not only because it is supposed to be, but because in the past that map may have helped you to get where you wanted to go. You trust the map, so you follow it. If you follow an accurate map, it will get you to your destination easily, without confusion. On the other hand, if you don't trust the directions, they can lead you in the wrong direction. If someone gives you directions on the side of the road, you may doubt the accuracy of the information. The directions may be perfectly accurate, but you doubt them, so you don't follow them exactly. Without both trust and accuracy, you can be led astray.

Examine Yourself to Find Your Way

You need to know how to live *now*. You can learn this information by finding your truth. Look deeply, and evaluate yourself honestly. Truly see the flaws and failures in yourself. Will your current belief system get you to a place of stable satisfaction? Has it helped you mature and function at a level that satisfies you? Have you seen some progress that indicates it is leading you to health and happiness?

The middle way is not a fad diet with a new twist or angle. The middle way is not a quick weight loss scheme. Reading this book also won't automatically make you fit. You have to do the work yourself, for no one else can do it for you. The middle way will help you open your eyes and your mind to see for yourself the reality of your situation and how you can achieve success in maintaining a healthy lifestyle, if you choose. The middle way means that you have to look at the reality of the facts and not make or take extreme dieting practices.

Many diet and exercise plans, books, pills, and equipment fail for a number of reasons. They aren't based on facts, so they do not help you get where you wanted to be. Any weight loss product that claims to be simple, easy, and quick is dishonest. When advertisers use these terms they only intend to sell the weight loss product. Their goal is not to help you. People will buy more if they believe it is easy and simple.

Successful living is not a destination on the map but a way of traveling—a way of living daily that brings you good health, well-being, and happiness. What kind of learning produces this successful way of living? Here are some guides:

- You can learn to alter your perspective to see that you can live a healthy, prosperous life today that will prepare you for a prosperous life for as long as you live.
- You can learn to change your old habits of automatically reacting reflexively without thinking.
- You can realign your perspective toward a reality that is consistent with being fit.
- You can learn the behaviors that give you brief satisfaction are not what make life worth living.
- You can learn that as much as there is pleasure in eating a chocolate cake, there can also be displeasure in it.

If you live a life based upon the middle way, you will learn that you can have a healthy, happy balance in your life. You can start changing what you have been told and think for yourself as you change to a more mature perspective.

Simple pleasures such as enjoying a chocolate cake are good, but without balance they can be harmful. The first step of the middle way is to realize that the map you've been following—the map that tells you chocolate cake is essential to enjoying life—is not accurate. Your life is worthwhile and pleasurable with or without cake.

Imagine a world where chocolate cake had never been invented. Your desire for cake could not exist, yet your life would go on quite well. Of course, the reality is chocolate cake does exist. Yet I hope you can begin to believe that if you never had another piece, you would not suffer a lesser quality of life. Whether or not eating cake affects you is determined by your mind and is a matter of perspective. You can decide not to have the desire to eat cake.

You have to learn not to trust the map that tells you to eat chocolate cake as a necessity for an enjoyable life. The easiest way of learning to view chocolate cake is to ignore it. If you don't put yourself in positions that will tempt your desires, those desires will not arise. As you advance and develop your maturity of mind, you will learn that you can exist in the room with the cake—you can see the cake and smell it and think about it—yet you will not accept it as an essential desire and will let any unwanted craving for it pass right by. Any desire to have cake is created in your mind. You have been taught it by common culture and you have learned it well. It is time to see the reality and rethink your map to living well.

You can further develop your maturity to see the chocolate cake from a perspective of balance in the middle way. You may decide that you want to taste the cake. You may conclude that having a little will add to the quality of your life at the moment, even though you could easily live without it. But thinking maturely, you would also decide that eating too much of that cake could harm you. With a balanced approach, you can come to know the correct amount to have. Too much can cause disharmony in your mind and body. Emotionally, you will regret having eaten too much, and physically you will have upset your digestion and narrowed your coronary arteries.

To make these decisions and all the others in your life, you can develop the mature adult within yourself. You can maintain conscious awareness of the choices you make. And you can use the reasoning powers within your mind.

As an example, imagine yourself at the carnival with a child. The child is overwhelmed with the desire to go on all the rides and can't think straight from all the excitement. The child wants to eat popcorn, candy apples, hotdogs, and on and on. As the adult, you are aware of the probable negative outcomes. You caution the child that he is likely to become sick from overeating.

When you as an adult ignore your conscious awareness, you can choose to overindulge in food. The child within you has taken over because you are not exercising mature control. You need the adult within you to remain aware to monitor the child within you continually.

Conscious awareness is the adult within you. Using this power of your mind, you will be better able to see the consequences of your actions before you take them. You will then be better able to make thoughtful, mature decisions that can lead to physical health and emotional happiness.

In the next chapter, I'll explain the reality of the relationship between metabolism and weight. As you have learned, they are related. They are also changeable.

Chapter 4

Metabolism and Weight

The Reality of Weight

You need food for nutrition, of course. But your body needs the right balance of the right variety of nutrition. You can have pizza, but if someone taller than you can eat two pieces and not gain weight, you can't necessarily afford to eat two pieces without risk of weight gain. You can have dessert, but do choose an appropriate portion for your body. Portions usually come in the same size, but the people who choose the portions are of different sizes.

As another example, a person who has a higher activity level can eat five or six cookies without risk of weight gain. A sedentary person, on the other hand, cannot eat that number of cookies without running the risk of gaining.

A taller person who is relatively more active has more body mass and burns more energy. This person needs to take in more food to maintain the body's structure, functions, and energy needs. No doubt you can fill in the blanks here: a shorter person who is more sedentary does not need as much food to maintain body structure, functions, and energy needs.

Metabolism refers to the burning of energy by the cells of a person's body, consuming or retaining as fat the energy from food. It is both a myth and a reality that skinny people are lucky to have high metabolism, whereas heavy people are fat because they have slow metabolism. Metabolism is partially a result of genetics and body type. Yet your metabolic level is primarily a result of the way you live. Your slow metabolism is a result of your low level of activity in comparison to the amount of food you eat.

Your metabolism is directly related to your activity level and your body mass. The two factors of activity level and body mass are controllable. You can become more active, and you can develop more muscle mass. That's the way you can change your metabolism. Fit people live a life that induces higher metabolism which keeps them fit. Heavy people live a life that is consistent with a slow metabolism causing them to be fat. You are rationalizing if you explain your obesity as a result of your slow metabolism. Be positive and realize that in fact you are choosing a lifestyle of slow metabolism which causes you to be overweight. You can change your lifestyle and develop a high metabolism and become fit.

You can also modify your metabolism by increasing your level of activity, the intensity of the activity, and the duration of the activity. In other words, you can exercise harder and longer. Furthermore, by altering your body proportions of fat and muscle, you can change your metabolism. More muscle activity means more metabolic reactions taking place. More muscle mass means metabolism happening at a higher rate.

Your mind decides what your body will eat and how active your body will be. If you are inactive, your body will have a lower metabolic rate, so you will not actively burn up the food you eat. If you are active, your body will have a higher metabolic rate and will actively burn up the food you eat.

As an analogy, consider a car idling at a stop light compared to a car on the highway going fifty miles an hour. The idling car burns fuel at a lower rate than the car going fifty miles an hour.

Your rate of metabolism also depends upon your body structure. In any activity, a taller person typically burns more calories than a shorter person in the same activity. The car analogy illustrates that different size cars will burn fuel at different rates as well. A heavier car will burn more of a given type of fuel than a lighter car will burn.

You cannot modify your stature, but you can keep metabolism in mind when you are figuring how much your body needs to eat. For instance, the body of a taller person usually needs more food than the body of a shorter person needs. The amount and duration of exercise each person does can influence the amount of food the body requires.

Your metabolism also depends on the composition of your body. A body that has more muscle mass than fat mass will have a higher metabolic rate. A body with more muscle mass has a higher metabolic rate because muscles actively burn calories.

Given all this information about height, activity, and body composition, how do you achieve the ideal weight for yourself? The answer lies in an equation—nothing difficult, I assure you.

The equation for your ideal weight is simple: it's a function of how much you eat and how much activity you perform. Without going into too much detail, a calorie is a measure of energy. You probably know that our bodies ingest calories in the form of proteins, carbohydrates, and fats. All of these elements are healthy and necessary for good nutrition. Fats are important for hormonal health and cell wall health. Carbohydrates are important for the fuel of your body to function. Proteins are important for maintaining muscles and the structural integrity of your body.

But a person should be careful not to choose too many foods from any one of these sources of calories. Lets consider for a moment, that we measure our food in the grams that scientists often use. A gram of fat usually packs in more calories—that is, energy—than a gram of carbohydrate or a gram of protein. Therefore, if you intend to lose weight, you should avoid choosing too high a proportion of your food from fats. Carbohydrates can stimulate your hunger, so you should avoid choosing carbohydrates as too high a proportion of your food. Also, too much protein can cause kidney problems, so you should avoid choosing proteins in too-high amounts.

You can see that all three types of nutrients—fats, carbohydrates, and proteins—can be both beneficial and detrimental, depending on your weight goals and on your need for nutrition. Keep in mind that there are no good calories or bad calories. And remember that your activity level determines how much calories your body burns.

Using the energy in calories—that is, burning those calories—can be achieved in various ways. You need not necessarily conjure images of grueling exercise accompanied by sweat and gasping. Any activity will burn calories. The more active and vigorous your activity, the more effectively you will burn calories. A sedentary way of living without much activity burns few calories and can cause your muscles to waste away, your bones to become brittle, and your heart and lungs to become unconditioned.

The weight you choose to be is within your control. You can select the amount and types of food that go into your body, as well as the type and level of activity that you will do. The final result is your responsibility.

The Weight Formula

What is the weight formula, and how can it work for you? The weight formula is a concept that depicts a way for you to understand how what you eat and how much you exercise will influence your body weight. It is not meant to be a complex calculable formula for our purposes but to help you understand the concepts relating food intake and exercise with weight. The weight formula indicates that the more you eat and drink, the more you will weigh if activity stays the same. Conversely, the higher your activity level, the lower you will weigh if food consumed stays the same. If you can keep food intake and activity the same, your weight will be stable. If you eat less, you are likely to lose weight over time. If you are more active, you are likely to lose weight over time.

Amount and types of food and drink = Weight
Amount and types of activity

If you enjoy being more analytical then please read on to the next section which goes into more detail. In any event, focus mostly on the concepts illustrated rather than getting overwhelmed by the mathematical type formula.

The Weight Formula in Depth

There are nine general combinations of food intake and activity. For each of these combinations, the relative amount of food/drink intake and the relative level of activity have a probable effect on body weight. These combinations are summarized in Table 1 and are explained in more detail in the discussion below.

Type 1)	High food and drink = Weight stable
High activity level

This person eats a large amount of food and exercises regularly and strenuously. Because the level of food intake and the activity level are in balance, the person's weight typically remains the same.

Type 2)	High food and drink = Weight gain
Moderate activity level

This person eats a lot of food and is active at work. The person occasionally does some exercise but does not exercise regularly. As a result, the person gains weight gradually. This person exercises sometimes but continues to eat more than the activity level justifies.

Type 3)	High food and drink = Weight gain
Low activity level

This person eats a lot of food and is sedentary, with minimal activity. As a result, the person gains weight gradually. It really doesn't matter if this person eats healthy types of food or not. The amount of food is too high for the level of inactivity, and weight gain results.

Type 4)   Moderate food and drink = Weight loss
High activity level

This person eats moderately and exercises strenuously. As a result, the person will gradually lose weight.

Type 5)   Moderate food and drink = Weight stable
Moderate activity

This person eats a moderate amount of food and exercises moderately, though not necessarily every day. Because the person's level of food intake and activity level are in balance, the person's weight typically remains the same.

Type 6)   Moderate food and drink = Weight gain
Low activity level

This person eats a moderate amount of food and is almost completely inactive. The activity level is not high enough to burn the energy produced by even a moderate diet. Weight gain is the result.

Type 7)   Low food and drink = Weight loss
High activity level

This person experiences rapid weight loss because the food intake is restricted and the person undertakes a high level of activity. The person has to be careful not to take either food restriction or exercise to unhealthy extremes. When this person reaches goal weight, s/he can increase food and drink to a moderate level and can decrease activity to a moderate level (as in Type 5). Using that approach, the person can maintain the goal weight.

Type 8)   <u>Low food and drink</u> = Weight loss
          Moderate activity level

          This person uses diet control accompanied by moderate exercise to lose weight gradually. After the person reaches goal weight, s/he can increase the food intake level to moderate and continue the moderate level of exercise to maintain a stable weight (as in Type 5).

Type 9)   <u>Low food and drink</u> = Weight stable
          Low activity level

          This person eats a small amount of food and rarely exercises. This person may not enjoy exercising or may be physically unable to exercise. Because the person's level of food intake and activity level are in balance, the person's weight typically remains stable.

As you continue reading and as you consider your own choices of amounts of food and drink to consume and your usual levels of activity, I encourage you to refer to this discussion as a guide. The choices you make will have a definite effect on your body weight. Changing those choices can change the effect.

Table 1. Weight Effects Expected from Food and Activity Combinations
(Numbers in parentheses refer to combination types discussed in the text.)

		Food and Drink Intake Levels		
		High	*Moderate*	*Low*
Activity Levels	*High*	(1) Weight stable	(4) Weight loss	(7) Weight loss
	Moderate	(2) Weight gain	(5) Weight stable	(8) Weight loss
	Low	(3) Weight gain	(6) Weight gain	(9) Weight stable

Chapter 5

The Mind Diet

The mind diet helps you become more aware of why, when, how much, and what you eat. With this information, you can better control your food intake. You can also start to relearn appropriate ways to think about food. We can start by examining some misguided notions about food and eating. We can develop rational awareness, knowing what we are doing before we do it. Please consider your answers to these queries:

- Why are you eating? Are you hungry when you are eating?
- When do you eat? Why do you eat at particular times? Is your decision to eat at a certain time automatic?
- How much food do you eat? Why do you eat as much as you do? Do you automatically eat a specific amount? Do you need to eat as much as you do? Do you eat more than really satisfies your hunger? Do you overeat to the point that the brief pleasure of eating is overshadowed by a longer period of feeling stuffed and tired?
- What foods do you choose to eat for each of your meals? Why are you eating particular foods? Are you avoiding other types of foods? If you do avoid certain foods, why do you avoid them? Have you tried all the foods available to you?

Few people have thought much about these questions. Most people do not see the reality of their eating. They do not maintain mature awareness of that reality. When you can see the reality of your actions, you can relearn and change your perspective of what you think about eating and food. Then you can achieve good balance in your life.

Healthy Food Tastes Good

Why do you eat certain types of foods? You have learned most of your beliefs about food from your family, your culture, and the media. You have learned to think certain foods are the most satisfying ones. But there is no basis in reality for your thinking. You believe that only certain and typically unhealthy foods give you satisfaction. Of course, variety in food is pleasurable, and it is reasonable to enjoy all types of food, whether the foods are healthy or not. Fit people can enjoy hamburgers, pizza, and ice cream. When you lose weight, you will enjoy those foods, too. But greasy, fatty, high carbohydrate meals are not the only types of food available. Healthy foods can be satisfying as well.

Every culture has its perspective on what is delicious, some of which other cultures may find revolting. As an example, Americans of fifty years ago would never have considered eating raw fish. The idea was disgusting. However, raw fish is extremely popular today and has several fancy names, including sushi, sashimi, and seviche.

These examples show that the mindset of some people and some cultures has changed its perspective. Raw fish can taste good to some but not to others. Whether you wish to eat raw fish depends upon your perspective. Any particular type of food that you may crave is not by its very nature delicious. Its appeal to you generally depends on how you were raised and how you now view that food in your mind. The way a food tastes is not a fixed characteristic of the food. Taste is the sensation in your mind.

Regardless of what you have thought about certain kinds of food, you can shift your perspective by rational thought. You can learn to genuinely appreciate healthier types of foods prepared in healthier ways.

With rational consideration, you can start to see that you can satisfy your hunger with almost any type of food. You can satisfy that food desire with healthy food just as easily as you can with unhealthy food. You might prefer to eat the foods that you have become accustomed to. But to satisfy your food needs, you can consciously plan to eat a healthy meal, finish that meal, and have your hunger satisfied.

Furthermore, you can gradually change your perspective as you learn to find tasty satisfaction in healthy foods as well. You have been culturally conditioned to think that only certain foods are tasty. You have learned that happiness results from eating large fatty carbohydrate meals. Yet you do not have to eat only advertised foods to be happy.

You probably realize that life is really not as completely blissful as some food commercials promise. Food companies want to sell a product, and their business goal is fair. It is also fair for you to realize that promises in commercials don't necessarily reflect reality. They create the need by creating the impression that buying and eating that food product will make you happy. Conversely, the culture starts to believe that without it life would be less pleasurable. You probably wouldn't buy an infomercial gadget that you really don't need. Yet the idea of the magical value of food to satisfy desire is so entrenched in our culture that many people believe it. When people around you believe in that magic, you may find it hard to see the truth.

Fast food restaurants should not be blamed for making people fat. When you have a meal at a fast food restaurant, you can make wise choices. You have free will to decide what you will eat. McDonalds doesn't force you to eat a Double Quarter-Pounder with cheese and to super-size your fries and drink. Though the marketing messages of such companies may try to urge you to eat large quantities, you as an intelligent, mature adult can choose the healthier options like salads and grilled chicken sandwiches without mayonaise. After you lose the weight, you can enjoy a Quarter-Pounder on occasion.

Are you Hungry When You Eat

Why do you eat? You eat because you need food to sustain yourself. Your body has evolved a complex neurological network to stimulate your brain with messages of hunger. Without the drive to eat, you would waste away. Your body should tell you when it needs refueling, not the clock. If you eat by the clock and not when your body tells you to, you are overeating.

If you ate too much at lunch and are still full by the usual time for dinner, you don't have to eat another meal. Wait until you get hungry. Wait until your body gives you the signal that it needs fuel. If you do not wait, you're eating for emotional or habitual reasons. Realizing this truth may help you to shift your perspective.

When you eat without having first felt hungry, you are denying yourself a simple, satisfying pleasure in life. You have not realized that you can increase the pleasure of any meal by being hungry before you begin eating. You are starting to become aware that eating as often as you can does not bring you as much pleasure as you thought. It is healthier to eat only when hungry and fortunately it will also bring you more pleasure, not less.

Imagine the truly deep satisfaction of being able to eat and enjoy your food with simple pleasure. You'll experience no guilt of needing to lose weight. Being fit and healthy brings you an incredible feeling about eating and enjoying many foods that you may not have chosen before. Your digestion will function better, and your meal is unlikely to upset your stomach or give you heartburn.

An overweight person usually can't enjoy a meal with pure pleasure because of guilt about needing to lose weight. If you are overweight, you may not even be hungry when you eat, and you waste an opportunity to enjoy the full pleasure of the meal.

Eating Healthy Is Happy

I hope you are starting to see the reality that eating and being healthy are more pleasurable than overindulging in food. I'd like you to realize, too, that if you take huge bites of your food, you lose the opportunity to enjoy the food. If you take smaller bites and slow down, you can enjoy the pleasure of the flavor and the satisfaction of eating more. Instead of taking huge bites that fill your mouth, take smaller bites. Large bites do not taste any better to your taste buds than smaller bites. Eating smaller amounts in each bite will automatically give you many more opportunities for tasting pleasure. If each small bite is half the size of a huge one, you will at least double the total number of bites for the same size meal. Just think! You'll have twice as many times to enjoy the flavor of the food and savor the satisfaction of eating. This way of eating is also healthier because it will allow you to eat more slowly and calmly, giving you more time to feel full and preventing you from overeating.

In addition to the size of the bite you can alter the composition of the item. For example, a peanut butter sandwich could be slightly fattening or excessively fatting simply by manipulating the amount placed on the sandwich. Reducing the amount of peanut butter in half doesn't reduce the taste satisfaction at all. Once you have stimulated all of your taste buds any other additional volume doesn't even contact your taste buds. Any additional peanut butter on the sandwich is a missed opportunity to enjoy the taste and only places unappreciated calories into your body.

Instead of taking in one bite immediately after the other, slow down to give yourself time for the pleasure of eating. If you slow down the rate at which you eat, you can double the time for chewing and tasting your food. Savor the food, enjoying its pure pleasure. Toss out your old ideas about getting in as much as you could. Eating thoughtfully and more slowly is healthier because it is better for good digestion and will lead you to eat only an appropriate amount.

Eating Less is More Pleasurable

Why do you eat more than you need? Without conscious awareness of what you are doing, the immature part of your mind gets triggered, and you forget logic and reason. I'd like for you to realize that if you eat until your stomach feels full and signals your brain to stop, it is too late. You have already overeaten.

When you maintain conscious awareness and think about enjoying food rather than eating as fast as you can, you will gain happiness and health. Think about how much you need to eat to satisfy your hunger. Decide before you eat how much you will eat—and then stop! Stop before you feel full. Stop before you finish all the food on your plate.

Sounds scary, doesn't it? You may not be able to imagine the thought of stopping before you feel full. But take a minute to rethink what you believe. If you eat the correct amount for your body, you will feel satisfied. Your satisfaction may take another thirty to sixty minutes, but if you ate the correct amount, you will feel satisfied.

Eating consistent types and sizes of meals will let you learn the appropriate, minimum amount you need to eat to bring on satiety thirty to sixty minutes after you have eaten. If a certain amount of food is making you feel very full or even bloated after you finish it, decrease the amount you choose to eat. Adjust the amount based on how you feel later. Also consider how you felt for the rest of the day. Did you function well with a smaller portion than you originally thought you needed? Adjust your food amounts until you find the right amount to give you enough to relieve your hunger.

Eating healthy will give you more happiness than overeating ever does. When you eat until your stomach tells you to stop, you have eaten too much. And what happens to that extra food? The excess calories will be deposited in your coronary and cranial arteries, clogging them and damaging the blood flow to your brain and heart. By overeating, you can physically damage yourself. You will also be unhappy because your stomach is uncomfortably full, preventing you from achieving a contented, balanced life. Remember to eat the right amount for your body and your emotional well-being.

When you overeat, the damage continues in a vicious cycle. Your digestive system goes into overdrive and pumps out excess insulin into your bloodstream. Then your blood sugar drops excessively, in turn stimulating the hunger response. As an example, imagine that you have just eaten a huge pasta meal. Then two hours later, you suddenly feel hungry again! "I just ate!" you scream inside, "so how can I possibly be hungry?"

It doesn't seem logical that you could be hungry again. Your body certainly isn't wasting away from lack of food. When you see the reality of physiology, you understand that your body works as it does. The vicious cycle may continue when you receive the low-blood-sugar message that you're hungry and need to eat again. Yet, with your new perspective, you can stop this awful, deadening cycle of hunger followed by bloating followed by more hunger. You have the power, and you can make the change.

Culture and Perspective on Fat and Fit

Eating healthy brings happiness. I urge you to ignore our culture's weaknesses. Think for yourself, and get happy. The culture argues that you should have big portions and go back for seconds to live a full and happy life. Start to think for yourself and see the reality that a fat, unhealthy culture dictates these "norms."

When you start getting more happiness from your life and eat appropriately, you may start to be noticed. The fat people will put pressure on you to join them in their unhealthy way of life. Yet you will be strong enough to maintain your conscious awareness of reality, and you will happily avoid being sucked into their false beliefs about food.

When you finally become healthy, some people may say you're too skinny. If you hear those remarks, see your doctor and get a second opinion. If you are too skinny, listen to the doctor. Extreme thinness will cause other health problems, both physical and emotional. People who develop an eating disorder such as anorexia may not realize they are sick. I urge you to have your physician involved and monitoring your health. If your doctor says you're not too skinny, ignore all the fat people who criticize you. They are speaking from their distorted perspective. You have the perspective that counts because you have opened your eyes to see the truth and made healthy changes.

Hunger in Your Stomach Not Your Brain

You have to learn the difference between real hunger and the desire just to eat. Real hunger is when you feel it in your stomach. Your stomach is legitimately empty sending you signals of real hunger. False hunger is when you feel it in your head with desire. Eat only when your stomach is truly hungry, not when you feel like eating for pleasure, lethargy or emotional reasons.

Think about the times when you have clearly eaten enough. Your stomach is full, and you no longer feel physically hungry—yet you still have an intense desire to eat. The next step for you in changing to a healthy perspective is to learn the difference between emotional hunger and physical hunger.

Emotional hunger is a desire to eat because you want to have a happy experience. Emotional hunger makes you want to eat to help yourself feel better. Emotional hunger often arises when you are stressed, depressed, or bored. Emotional hunger urges you to eat because you "deserve" a reward. Emotional hunger is eating because you are tired.

You can control your emotional hunger with the power of your intelligent mind. Keep that false hunger in check by thinking about whether you really need to eat. Can you wait a little longer and not suffer? If you can put off eating until you are really hungry, you will be in control.

Suppose you slip and start eating without thinking first whether your hunger is emotional or real. Don't worry—it is never too late to regain control of yourself. Even if you have eaten half a piece of cake, you can stop and throw the rest away. Don't rationalize that you've already eaten half, so you might as well finish the rest of the cake. Emotional hunger does matter at any time. If you don't eat the remaining half, you have succeeded in eliminating half the intake of calories from that cake. You are in control again.

Never rationalize that you'll just start over tomorrow or next week. Why wait? You have the opportunity now to do something about it. Why make weight loss harder on yourself? Why pile on more work for you to do next week? It is far easier to stop and gain control even in mid-bite than it is to let the pounds add up to be dealt with later. Starting to gain control next week will be harder than simply starting now.

Waiting involves rationalizing and not accepting the reality of your situation. With practice and mental awareness, changing your perspective and your eating behavior will be easier for you.

Strengthen Your Awareness

As you develop your mind and body, you will use all that you have learned mentally and physically. You can apply this information to every situation as you continue to control your mind and desires. Remember that the choices are all in your power. You have to make your mind and your body do what you want.

I suggest practicing this power by buying a large portion of your favorite unhealthy food. Put the food in front of you, and leave it there for the entire day. At the end of the day, eat half the portion. Leave the other half there until the next day, and then throw it away. (Obviously, if your favorite unhealthy food requires refrigeration or freezing, you will take those steps.)

Variations of this mental exercise can help you develop the strength in your mind to be mentally aware of your emotions and your desires. You will always be faced with choices, and you can learn to make the right choices. The temptations will be all around you. With an intelligent, conscious approach, you can control your desires.

First, you should realize that a desire is just that—a desire—and it does not have to be satisfied. If a pie is on the table, the pie is not in control. You are. You can live a happy life without eating the pie. If you eat the pie, the satisfaction will be brief, but the mental anguish and guilt from overeating will last far longer. Most of all, you will regret losing control of yourself.

Ultimately, the pie will bring you more dissatisfaction than pleasure. Why make yourself suffer for a few fleeting minutes of superficial pleasure? Without balance, you will find yourself in a vicious cycle of desire followed by false promises unrealized. Eating in an unhealthy way is not really fun and does not give you lasting happiness. Life has many more satisfying pleasures to offer. Find happiness in the rest of your life. Don't be so simple as to believe that eating is your main pleasure.

When you follow the middle way and maintain conscious awareness, you can make decisions that will bring you happiness. Put the mature adult within you up on your shoulder to watch over you. You know the truth, and you just need to remind yourself all the time.

- Eat healthy food because it tastes good.
- Eat healthy amounts because a reasonable level of satiety is more pleasurable than upsetting your stomach.
- Eat healthy because you will live longer and give yourself more chances to eat in the future.

Remember that the healthy person will enjoy food more than the unhealthy ones. After you lose the weight, you will be a healthy person. Then you can reap the benefits of being at your goal weight. These rewards are many and joyous!

- You can eat the way a fit person does and enjoy all the pleasures of a balanced way of living.
- You will enjoy all the foods that life has to offer.

- You will approach food with a rational, balanced approach.
- You will eat anything you desire, good or bad, but not too much of anything.

In your first phase of weight loss, you will learn many things that will make you an expert in becoming thin. This first phase, however, requires putting yourself in a state of imbalance. You will have to eat less food than you burn in activity. After you lose the weight, you can eat food that equals what you burn in activity.

Losing weight will seem hard at first, but as you have success, your increased motivation and happiness will make the process easier. Start with conscious awareness, and maintain it to eat right.

Chapter 6

The Practical Diet

The middle way is based on the principle of a balanced life. Unfortunately, if you are overweight, you are out of balance. In order to achieve a healthy way of living, you can choose to live out of balance in the other direction to lose the weight. After you reach the right weight for your body, maintaining a balanced life will be much easier for you. The principles of the middle way will be clear to you by then, and you can occasionally turn to them on occasion so that you can maintain a healthy balance in your life and your food choices.

You may not necessarily find all of the tools effective for you. You may adopt some of the principles completely, and as you mature in your understanding, you may choose to alter them honestly to fit your situation.

After a while, you will become so skilled at losing weight that it may be difficult for you to readjust your way of living to the balanced one. After becoming so good at losing weight, you may have to relearn how to be in a steady state. You'll have to make sure that you don't become unbalanced in the opposite direction and grow too thin and unhealthy.

Conscious awareness and balance in your perception will be your guide to eating healthy. When you start to change the way you view food and eating, I hope you will realize that long-lasting happiness is not based on the food you eat. When an overweight person eats food, s/he is satisfying a want or desire that doesn't last beyond the meal. Without balance, such a person is locked in a vicious cycle of desire followed by false promises unrealized.

If you analyze this person's situation, you can see that eating unhealthy is not really fun and does not offer happiness. Eating healthy is much more satisfying through the perspective of the middle way. You know the truth, and you need to remind yourself of the reasons for eating healthy, according to the middle way:

- Eat healthy food because it does taste good.
- Eat healthy amounts because a reasonable level of satiety is more pleasurable than upsetting your stomach and digestion.
- Eat healthy food because it is good for you and will lead to many more opportunities to enjoy a longer and more functional life.
- Following the middle way will lead to many more enjoyable eating opportunities because you are likely to live longer than if you are obese.

The amount of time you spend eating and enjoying food is insignificant compared to what you do in the rest of your life. Conversely, the amount of time you may be thinking about eating is a waste of your valuable time. Learn to start thinking that your happiness and pleasure in life do not depend on what you eat. Food is simply necessary for supporting your physical body, nothing else.

Food enjoyment is a secondary benefit. You do not even have to enjoy the food you eat. You could eat simple, bland, boring food, yet your body would survive. Think about all the other things in your life that make your life satisfying. You can live happily without any of the products that marketers tell you are necessary. Fast food and beverage companies want you to buy their products. They hope to convince you and the rest of society that happiness is impossible for those who don't buy and consume what they're selling. But do you really believe that you have to buy and consume all the unhealthy products that have been marketed to you? See life more realistically than a series of exaggerated and blissful commercials. See the facts and use your conscious awareness to control what you think and feel. It is not easy. It takes practice.

Our culture has burdened the word *diet* with connotations of self-starvation, of not being permitted to eat as much as one wants, and of eating particularly untasty foods. The middle way approach to weight loss focuses as much on your mind as on what you eat. The middle way is not a quick-fix fad. It is based upon realistic principles. As you have probably learned from experience, there is no easy way to erase weight.

In following the middle way, try to stop believing that people are fat or fit naturally. Fit people can become fat. Fat people can become fit. Either condition is not permanent and can be changed. Fat people are not naturally overweight, but they eat more than they burn. Fit people are not thin naturally, but they burn what they eat.

People's body sizes are based on simple mathematics and chemical reactions in the body. I ask you to stop listening to the lie that you will get fat as you get older because your metabolism "slows down". You metabolism isn't slowing down. The only thing slowing down is yourself, your mind, and what you will your body to do. Plenty of older people are not fat because they have not allowed themselves to eat too much or to slow down in their activities.

This myth of thinness only for youth falls apart as we take a closer look. It used to be that young people were predominantly thin. Children would play all day and ate a lot to support their activity, but never got fat. Then those children grew up and sit around at a desk all day, eating doughnuts and big lunches. Are you surprised that these formerly thin children grew fat?

Adults don't have slow metabolism. They just become less active and eat too much for their reduced level of activity. Today, children are fat for the same reason. They are not very active, and they eat more junk food. Thin adults are not naturally thin. They are more physically active in proportion to the calories they eat.

Practical Diet Ideas

Sometimes, especially when you're losing weight, you'll need techniques that are appropriate for weight loss. However, some of these approaches are clearly out of balance with the middle way. Please understand that these techniques are for temporary use during your weight loss period. Some of these methods can be modified to be less extreme after you have achieved your goal weight and will fit into your healthy life.

When you're focused on losing weight and reaching your goal weight, learning to deal with temptations is crucial. Don't go to the places that you know will challenge you to overeat. Wait to go to those places until you have better learned to deal with such challenges. The most important place this applies is your home. Make your list of grocery items and stick to the list. Never go grocery shopping on an empty stomach. If you get carried away at the grocery store and buy too much food or the wrong foods, have someone else do the shopping. Alternatively, you can shop online to avoid temptation. Remember that the foods you bring into your house will be the foods that will tempt you. When you have limited choices in the house, you will automatically be restricted in what you can eat. For a snack, your only options available will be healthy items.

Over time, by necessity, you will change your perspective on eating. You will come to appreciate healthier food. You will learn to appreciate the natural flavors as your tastes gradually change. You will slowly realize that you can survive without junk foods and other unhealthy foods. You will build an awareness of the other parts of your life that bring you satisfaction.

When you make a meal for dinner, make just enough to eat. Don't bring serving trays to the dinner table with extra rolls, for example. If you bring extra food to the table, you will be more tempted to eat it while you are still waiting for your feeling of satisfaction from the meal to set in.

If you do make extra food, don't bring it to the table. Serve the plates with the planned portions, and set them on the table. Don't tempt yourself at the table. Similarly, don't linger at the table after you have eaten, especially if there is food sitting in front of you. Get up from the table, and go do something. Make yourself get out of the kitchen and the temptation zone. If you do wish to stay at the table for social purposes, make sure you have cleared away the food.

You can also control what you eat when you are at work. Bring your lunch to work. Plan ahead, and prepare the lunch with awareness of its health value. If you go out to lunch, you will be challenging yourself and you may not be mentally ready. Don't put yourself in those positions that tempt you. If you do eat out or at a cafeteria, select consistent meals from day to day, so that you can learn how much will be enough to fill you. Try not to order different types of meals because it will be hard for you to know the right amount to eat. Later, when you have learned well, you will have good judgment on the similarity of different meals to satisfy you.

It is all right to eat in your car, especially if you have thoughtfully planned and selected your breakfast meal on the road to be nutritionally appropriate, there will be no temptations to order more or to eat incorrectly. You will be forced to eat what you brought and will be forced not to overeat because nothing else is readily available. Eating in your car is an efficient use of your time and will help make time for your other activities, including exercise.

It is all right for fit people to eat before going to bed because they won't eat for a full six to eight hours. If you are not hungry before breakfast, you may have eaten too much the night before. Thin people can enjoy guilt-free snacks before bed. However, snacking late at night is not a good idea while you are trying to lose weight.

Wherever you are and whatever size portion you are served, you can consciously remind yourself that you do not have to eat the entire portion. Don't automatically go into eating mode, intending to clear the plate. Decide in advance what you reasonably know is the right portion, and eat only that much. By slowing your mind and thinking like a mature, rational adult, you can consciously decide how much of the food to eat.

Keep your body and mind busy to avoid boredom. When your body gets lethargic or your mind gets bored, you will falsely have the sense that you need to eat to energize yourself. If you occupy your mind and body with other activities, there will be less time for your mind to be tempted. When the body and mind are not active, there is no stimulus to maintain higher energy levels. When you are active, the body is stimulated, and energy chemicals are triggered to maintain a vigorous level of energy. When you are sedentary you will inevitably become lethargic because your body has no stimulus to be awake. You will feel as though you need to eat to give you energy. This is a false sense of hunger. Your body is not hungry, but is tired from lack of activity. The best solution is to become more active to stimulate your body to wake up. Becoming more active will stimulate your body so that you will feel awake and have more energy.

As an example, when you leave your car sitting in the driveway, it takes a while for the temperature to rise so that the engine can run at full speed. If the car has been running recently, it will still be warm and starts up more quickly and reaches full speed sooner. Similarly, your body has a natural ability to do what you ask it to do. When you lie around too long, the body starts to slow down, as if it thinks it is time to sleep. Activity tells your body to be in awake mode and stimulates it to be energetic. Inactivity tells the body it is time to go to sleep and shuts off the stimulus for energy.

The body has a natural feedback mechanism that you can use to your advantage. With a lower energy level, you may falsely have the sense to eat to give yourself energy. Stay active to increase your energy level, and you won't eat unnecessarily.

Controlling your appetite and feeling satisfied after meals will be hardest in the beginning of your weight loss. Your stomach is stretched out and has been trained by overeating to be able to take in large volumes of food. As your stomach gets smaller, it will begin to give you a satisfied feeling much sooner, and the satisfied feeling will last longer. When your stomach is smaller, you will find it easier to achieve your weight goals. You will feel perfectly content after a reasonable meal. This feeling of contentment will last for a longer time. Between meals, you will not feel hungry all the time.

Eventually, you will be eating smaller meals more frequently. This approach is the healthiest way to feed your body. You can maintain a more level, steadier amount of insulin. You will avoid large fluctuations in your blood sugar level, creating a healthier body and reducing the frequency of hunger.

Eating multiple smaller meals has numerous benefits. You will reverse the trend of distending you stomach with larger meals and will stimulate your stomach to begin contracting. This is like a nonsurgical stomach stapling or gastric bypass. Your stomach will get smaller, like a thin person's stomach, and you will become full faster than a fat person with a large stomach does.

Amazingly, you will be growing slimmer and will be eating more frequently than you did when you were fat! As a slimmer person, you will have more episodes during the day to feel the enjoyment of eating—up to five or six times a day. Although the meals will be smaller, they will be completely satisfying to you. You will not overeat. You will be patient and wait for a sense of satiety to come over you.

Fat Deposition Control

Realize that eating less frequently and in larger portions throughout the day stimulates your body to deposit fat. This happens for two reasons. Excess calories that the body cannot use immediately will be stored as fat. Furthermore, less frequent meals signal your body that the food supply is infrequent and stimulates your body to deposit fat to give energy between the meals.

Furthermore, eating smaller meals spread throughout the day will also affect your metabolism by controlling fat deposition. Our bodies have evolved to deposit fat if it believes that meals are sporadic as in times of famine. So when you have longer gaps between meals the body will tend to deposit fat in storage because it may need the calories before the next meal. When you eat frequently your body learns that it will be getting necessary calories regularly. There is no stimulus to deposit fat because meals are frequent, supplying the calories necessary to fuel the body for the next few hours until the next meal.

When you eat more than a reasonable amount at any one sitting, your body will automatically store those extra calories as fat. Also, when you do it regularly, your body gets really good at depositing fat. Your body knows it will get more food than it needs, so it becomes a fat-depositing machine. This fat-reserve process is part of our genetic protectiveness from a time when food was not always available. When meals were plentiful, the body would deposit fat in order to have sufficient reserves for energy to get through the times when food was scarce. Even with today's plentiful food, your body still thinks it should store excess food as fat. When you eat excessively on a regular basis, your body becomes even better at converting the extra food into fat.

As an illustration, if you were to wait all day without eating and ate 2,000 calories at dinner you would deposit more fat than if you ate 2,000 calories by 5 meals of 400 calories spread throughout the day. The long period of time without food tells your body that food is scarce and the next time it receives excess it is planning to store some as fat for the next time there is a long gap without food. Furthermore, the body can only use so much fuel to function at that time and so all the excess is automatically deposited as fat. Be very careful to realize eating more frequently you will have to be vigilant to limit the quantity you eat to a reasonable portion.

Understand and Accept Hunger

When you're on the middle way diet, you will have to deal with hunger, and hunger can certainly be emotionally challenging. It should help you if you remember that this weight-loss period is temporary and will end when you have achieved the appropriate weight. After you reach your goal, you can live and eat more naturally. Use this knowledge to realize that the hunger stress will pass.

In order to lose weight, you will have to deprive yourself of satiety to some degree. Find comfort in the knowledge that when you are feeling hungry, you are losing the weight. If you feel hungry, the hunger offers emotionally positive feedback that you are accomplishing your weight-loss goal. If you feel so hungry that you can't wait until the next meal, on occasion it is all right to have a tiny snack, though not enough to fill your stomach.

Disregard the natural urge to eat may seem impossible. The good news is that you also know how to disregard these urges. In the beginning of weight loss, the urges are most intense, but if you use your mental conscious awareness and ignore those intense temporary feelings, they will pass. Your nervous system will adapt to the feeling of hunger, and the signals will gradually diminish. You will not get hungrier and hungrier.

After a few days, you will learn to find pleasure in the knowledge that you're achieving progress. Your success can further motivate you, and you will enter a success cycle rather than the vicious cycle of eating and getting fat.

Eat the same meals regularly to help you learn the amount that will reasonably satisfy you. Eat the same breakfast and lunch as much as you can. By "the same," I mean reasonably similar. Lunch sandwiches can vary from meat to meat types. But avoid hard to compare meals, such as eating spaghetti and meatballs one day and steak another day. By keeping the meals consistent, you will learn the right volume to eat to reasonably satisfy your hunger. If you eat different meals every day, you'll have more difficulty knowing how much food is enough. When you get thinner, you can add some variety to your meals.

Eating consistent types of meals will also help you learn how much you need to eat to lose weight. If you are eating consistent but not losing weight, clearly you have overestimated. You need to cut back on the amount of food. Since you have been eating similar meals, you can figure more easily how much to cut back.

You can start by cutting back on the portion size by making conscious, planned decisions, such as taking a slice of bread off your regular sandwich. Over time, these reductions will make a difference. You may consider eating half a banana with your breakfast instead of a whole banana. By having a routine meal, you have a standard by which you fine-tune to your needs.

Increasing your activity level is also helpful in weight loss. If you are consistent in your eating habits and activity levels, you will know exactly how to tweak your plan to get results. After you have lost weight, you can make adjustments in either direction to maintain a healthy weight.

It is not advisable to be a strict calorie counter in the sense of adding up each individual item and continuously fixating on your calorie intake. It is not reasonable to live this way in the long term. Fit people don't live this way. The demands of the calorie-counting approach are too strict and difficult to manage. You should, however, have some basic idea of the contents of the foods you are eating. Knowing that information, you will be able to have consistency in your diet by making similar substitutions. For instance, if you normally have a banana with breakfast, you know that an apple has similar content and would be a good substitute. If you have no idea of what you are eating, you may be susceptible to choosing an item with a higher calorie count.

If you find yourself in a situation that requires you to veer away from your planned diet, you can make a conscious decision to eat half what you would normally eat in that situation. For example, if you find yourself with people who want to get ice cream, and if you want to enjoy some ice cream with them, order half the amount you would normally order on such an occasion. If you would normally get a double scoop, get a single scoop. If you usually eat whole-milk ice cream, you may find that ice milk is available. While not as rich-tasting as ice cream, the ice milk will allow you a small indulgence and still not pull you too far off your planned program.

You can also avoid temptation when you're dining away from home. Don't eat the bread on the table before the meal. Don't order an appetizer. Instead, order a protein-rich dish with vegetables for fiber, and enjoy it. You will probably be very satisfied and still feel good physically and emotionally. Your pleasure in eating with friends will not turn into a feeling of guilt over eating too much or eating the wrong foods.

It is never too late to stop eating a dish or a serving. You don't have to finish just because you started it. You may rationalize that you have failed to remain on your planned program and say to yourself, "Oh, I might as well finish this off and start my diet again later." This approach is self-defeating. Just because you have eaten half an unhealthy food does not mean you have failed your program. The opportunity to succeed begins is at the moment you are deciding whether or not to finish the food. Even if you have already eaten almost all of the food, you will succeed if you do not finish it. Maybe the next time you are tempted, you will improve and will stop sooner—or preferably not start eating at all.

Always remember that it is never too late to start. Never put off an opportunity to be healthy and to reach your goals. Also, when you contemplate when to begin or resume your middle way program, for example, you can and should start it immediately. Any recent failure does not justify waiting until later to start again. Give yourself a break! If you fail one day, that lapse is not an automatic end and a permanent failure. It is a brief setback. Let it go, forgive yourself for being human, and start over as soon as possible.

Diets often fail because they are complicated, difficult-to-follow regimens not based on reason. They are cumbersome and hard to fit into your life. Fit people learn to think for themselves and make food selections based upon what they have learned. You should have balance in your meals. But don't make this weight loss process complicated. You should not spend too much, if any, time on counting calories or foods or pounds. Keep a general idea of what you are doing and eating, but don't get carried away with a calculator. Fit people do not live their lives constantly counting and adding up calories.

You can help yourself toward success if you simply read labels to learn about the foods you are eating. This process will help you learn which foods are healthy and appropriate. You want to know how much protein, fat, and carbohydrates are in each food you consider eating. Over time, you can easily know or predict what is in foods. By reading labels, you will gradually understand the total calories in a certain amount of a particular type of food. By learning how many calories are in an apple or banana, you will be able to make educated guesses about other fruits. Knowing how much fat is in a handful of peanuts, you will be able to make an educated guess about the fat content of almonds and other types of nuts.

Pre-packaged diet meals can be useful. Diet meals help you know exactly what you are eating—calories, protein, fat, and carbohydrates. These meals help to standardize your daily regimen so that you can make adjustments based on your personal needs. I caution you to make sure the diet meals are preservative-free. Also, make sure the portions are appropriate for you.

More Tips

Avoid letting your body stay too cold because you will have a stronger urge to eat a lot when you're cold. Hunger varies by seasons and body temperatures. In the winter, your body will tend to be hungrier than in the summer. When you are hot and uncomfortable in warm weather, you will have a smaller appetite. Furthermore, people tend to be more active in the warmer seasons stimulating increased metabolism. Consciously, be aware to plan activities during winter when we have a tendency to become inactive indoors.

Never buy larger-size clothes when your original-size clothes won't fit. Needing larger clothes is a clear sign that your weight needs control. Continue to wear the clothes you have so that you can remind yourself that you need to lose weight. If you accommodate the fat with larger clothes, you will allow yourself to feel comfortable and will permit yourself to continue gaining weight. If you continue to wear the clothes that are too small, you will feel tight and uncomfortable forcing you to make the necessary efforts. Tighter clothes in your waist will also make you feel fuller by putting pressure on your abdomen. Belt tightness can be used effectively to create a sense of fullness. Never increase your belt loop size. Leave it where it is even though it may feel uncomfortable. It will remind you of your size and of your need to lose the fat.

In the next chapter, I'll explain the ratio diet as an important way to achieve the balance required for living the middle way.

Chapter 7

The Ratio Diet

The middle way says that you should maintain a balance in the amounts of food you eat. The amount you eat should be appropriate for your weight and activity level. Furthermore, you need to balance the amounts of protein, fiber, carbohydrate and fat you eat. All these elements are crucial to a healthy diet. None should be eliminated, and none should be eaten exclusively, but you should eat them in reasonable proportions. The ratio diet will help guide you.

Protein is important and necessary for the structure of your body. It also increases the sense of fullness after meals. In general eat more protein. However, if you eat too much protein, you may risk kidney damage.

Fiber is important for gastrointestinal health. It also increases the sense of fullness after meals. In general eat more fiber. However, too much or too little fiber can have deleterious effects.

Water is important for hydration. It also is helpful to drink extra with meals to fill your stomach and satisfy your hunger.

Carbohydrates are important to fuel your body. They also tend to make you get hungry sooner after a meal so limit intake of carbohydrates to reasonable levels. If you eat too much in carbohydrates, you risk obesity and diabetes.

Fat is important and necessary for your body as well. If you don't eat enough fat, you risk having inadequate hormone levels. If you eat too much fat, you risk obesity, atherosclerosis, heart disease, and stroke.

Proteins

Most people do not eat enough protein. Their usual diet is so full of junk food, snack food, and soft drinks that it contains too little protein.

Protein is the building blocks of the body. It is part of all your cells, tissues, and organs, as well as your bones, muscles, and skin. Protein also forms your blood and its enzymes. You need protein for growth and for replacing the body cells that degenerate every day. Protein also is a significant part of your immune system.

Though protein can provide energy to your body, excess protein may be converted to fat and be stored in your body. Furthermore, excess protein intake may damage your kidneys. Diabetics should be particularly careful because their kidneys are susceptible to failure.

You can increase the amount of protein in your diet by eating more meats and fish. As much as possible, the meat you eat should be lean. Chicken, turkey breast, and other lean cuts, along with fish, offer excellent sources of protein. Almost any reasonably lean red meat such as filet mignon or low-fat ground meat is acceptable in reasonable amounts and frequency. Most meats are acceptable as long as they are not processed with extra fats or fried. Protein rich meats will create a longer lasting satisfaction to your hunger.

Meats give your body the protein necessary for building tissue and bone. High protein meals will truly satisfy your hunger. Include lean meats in most of your meals. The amount of protein you need depends on your weight and activity level—perhaps 60 to 120 grams a day. The average adult needs 0.45 mg per pound of body weight. An endurance athlete may need up to 0.7 mg per pound of body weight. A strength exercise athlete may need up to 0.8-1.0 mg per pound of body weight.

Since the average person needs .45 mg of protein per pound of body weight this can be approximated by rounding to .5 mg per pound. Therefore, you can easily calculate your minimum daily protein requirement by halving your body weight. For example, a 120 pound person would need a minimum intake of 60 grams of protein. A 150 pound person would need a minimum of 75 grams of protein. A 180 pound person would need 90 grams of protein.

I have developed the Protein Fat Ratio to help you select healthy protein meals that don't contain too many fat grams. The Protein Fat Ratio can be calculated by dividing the number of protein grams by the number of fat grams. This number will preferably be more than 3, but a result more than 2 is acceptable. If you are not making progress with your weight loss, be more aggressive and choose foods with a Protein Fat Ratio of more than 4 or 5.

As an example, half of a chicken breast with skin that has been dipped in batter and fried would have 35 grams of protein and 18 grams of fat. The protein grams (35) divided by the fat grams (18) equals 1.9—a result less than 3 and not preferable. Your goal for weight loss is to maximize protein grams and limit fat grams.

A better choice would be half of a chicken breast with skin roasted. The protein would be 29 grams and the fat would be 8 grams. The Protein Fat Ratio would be calculated as 29 protein grams divided by 8 fat grams equals 3.6, which is above 3 and preferable.

If you wanted to be more aggressive, you could eat half a roasted chicken breast without the skin. The Protein Fat Ratio would be calculated as 27 protein grams divided by 3 fat grams, and the result equals 9. This is an excellent index, well above the minimum of 3.

Fiber

You should try to eat about 25-30 grams of fiber each day, whether or not you are on a weight loss program. Most dietary fiber comes from vegetables, fruits, and whole grains. The two types of fiber are soluble and insoluble. Foods that have soluble fiber include legumes (such as beans, peas, and lentils), oatmeal, nuts, seeds, apples, pears, strawberries, and blueberries. Foods that have insoluble fiber include whole-grains (breads, bagels, hot and cold breakfast cereals, noodles, rice), wheat bran, and vegetables, especially cauliflower, broccoli, carrots, and cabbage. These foods also have a lot of carbohydrate, but they are good because they have high fiber content, which is necessary for your gastrointestinal system.

Increase fiber in your diet for health and to suppress hunger. You can find fiber in vegetable, grains and fruits. Select them in that order. Vegetables are high in fiber and should be a basic part of your meals. Other good fiber sources include beans, lentils, and legumes. High fiber grains are a better alternative to plain white rice and pasta. High fiber fruits such as apples are a great between meal snack.

You can also increase your water and fluid volume intake in order to avoid binding your bowels with dry fiber in your colon. Dietary fiber needs adequate amounts of water to keep digestion flowing. You should hope to have a bowel movement daily. You can expect to develop a daily toilet routine, particularly in the morning before you start your day. Early in the morning, your parasympathetic nervous system is active and stimulates your bowels to function while your body is inactive. After you start your day, your sympathetic nervous system is active, stimulating your body and suppressing your gastrointestinal system, thus reducing your opportunities for bowel movements.

High fiber and lots of water alone are not adequate to keep the gastrointestinal system working. Keep your body active to avoid constipation. A high fiber diet will help to prevent colon cancer and increases your sense of fullness. Higher fiber foods will make you feel full faster and for a longer period.

Fiber can be used in many ways. Eat high fiber and low sugar cereals for breakfast with nonfat milk. The fluid and fiber volume will help to fill your stomach and will satisfy your hunger. Eat whole grain breads with your sandwich at lunch. Eat high fiber vegetables with your dinner. If you need to snack between meals, think of high fiber fruits, but only when you have become fit. These fruits are higher in sugars and can be difficult to manage while you are trying to lose weight.

I have created the concept of Carbohydrate Fiber Ratio to help you select healthy high fiber meals without too much simple carbohydrates. It is important to eat fiber, and it is expected that carbohydrates come with most fiber foods. However, it is important not to take in too many carbohydrates to get the fiber.

The Carbohydrate Fiber Ratio can be calculated by dividing the number of carbohydrate grams by the number of fiber grams. Ideally, the Carbohydrate Fiber Ratio should be less than 10. On the other hand, if you are not losing weight, be more aggressive and eat foods producing a Carbohydrate Fiber Ratio of less than 9, 8, 7, 6, or even 5.

As an example, a slice of plain white bread may have 17 grams of carbohydrate and 1 gram of fiber. The Carbohydrate Fiber Ratio is calculated by dividing carbohydrate grams (17) by fiber grams(1). So 17 divided by 1 equals 17, which is not less than 10 and is not acceptable. Remember that a Carbohydrate Fiber Ratio of less than 10 maximizes fiber intake and limits carbohydrate intake.

A better choice would be a slice of whole grain bread that may have 20 grams of carbohydrate and 3 grams of fiber. The Carbohydrate Fiber Ratio would be calculated as 20 carbohydrate grams divided by 3 fiber grams equaling 6.6—a result less than 10 and acceptable.

Carbohydrates

The average person eats too many carbohydrates, which can contribute to obesity when eaten to excess. Reducing the volume of carbohydrates in your diet means eating less pasta, rice, bread, snack foods. For instance, when you have spaghetti and meatballs, cut back on the amount of spaghetti. Meals heavy in carbohydrates will cause a sharp increase in your blood sugar, stimulating your body to produce insulin that causes low blood sugar and feelings of hunger.

To reduce carbohydrates, you can also reduce the number of sweets and desserts. These foods will exacerbate weight gain and will make you even hungrier than if you had not eaten them.

All starches such as bread, pasta, and rice are converted into sugars. In selecting carbohydrates, choose healthy ones such as whole grain and high-fiber breads that are slower to be converted into sugar. Whole grain foods retain the healthy parts of the grain, and high fiber foods are less stimulating to your insulin levels.

Avoid drinking fruit juice or soda. Fruit juice is a lot like soda; it just has more vitamins which should be obtained from real fruit. Furthermore, soda companies are now marketing added vitamins to some of their product lines. You shouldn't believe that soda with vitamins added is healthy. Fruit juice is essentially the same. In the end they are both full of excess calories from sugar that will stimulate your hunger. Many people feel that since fruit juice is "good for you" that they can drink as much of it as they like. It is better to eat whole fruits that contain natural fiber that will satisfy your hunger compensating for the sugar. Whole fruits have the benefit of fiber and vitamins but have a high sugar content and could easily be abused like candy if not reasonably selected. After you have lost weight, you can choose to reincorporate small amounts of fruit juices into your diet.

You can easily reduce your carbohydrate intake. Eat fewer high-starch foods such as breads, pastas, rice, potatoes in any form, chips and snack foods when you are on the middle way weight reduction diet.

I make no specific recommendations on the amount of carbohydrate you should eat. How much you need depends on how fast you wish to lose weight. Also, the amount you need also depends on your activity level. If you are active and at goal weight, you will need more carbohydrates to fuel you body and its activities. Here are some ideas for reducing the carbohydrates in your meals.

- Remove one slice of bread from your sandwich, and eat that sandwich open-face. Make that slice of bread whole grain to increase the fiber in your diet.
- Eat half of a potato, without butter and sour cream.
- Cut the amount of rice in half, and use whole-grain, high-fiber rice.
- Make your pasta a side dish, not the main dish.

The sugar obtained naturally from fruits and eaten in reasonable, balanced portions is appropriate. Don't add sugar to any food, no matter what you are eating. Sugar, as I have said, is high in calories and creates more hunger. Do not eat sugar based foods such as candy, deserts, pies, cakes, doughnuts and even sugary coffee drinks—except in small amounts on special occasions.

Fats

The average person consumes more fat than the body needs. Most obese people need to reduce the fat in their diet. Any fats that are naturally a part of the food should not be feared. You need some fat in your diet so it might as well come as a part of the natural foods you eat. Fat is an excellent hunger satisfier because it creates a long-lasting sense of contentment.

Avoid nuts when trying to lose weight because of the high fat content. They are healthy and good for you only when you are fit. Otherwise, when you are fat, their health benefits are outweighed by the high fat content. You can also eat steak, which is high in fat but tastes good, and life is to be enjoyed.

On the other hand, you should not seek out extra fat. Concentrate on low-fat foods, but accept higher-fat food when it is part of protein rich meats. Under no circumstances should you have any fat that has been added to the food in preparation or in dressing the foods. Such oils and fats are unnecessary and, in the weight loss phase, off limits.

For example, do not add cheese to anything you eat. Why add several hundred calories and several dozen grams of fat to a food? By eliminating the cheese and mayonnaise from a sandwich, you can eat the same meal, eliminate unneeded fat and calories, and still enjoy the delicious taste. If you eat a steak, enjoy it without a creamy sauce. Enjoy the natural flavor of the meat without the extra oils.

Don't add oil to your food. Even the healthy oils are not really healthy when you add them to food unnecessarily. There is no good added oil, no matter what you may have heard. Oil is oil. Oil is fat. Fat is fat. Do not eat added oil and believe that it is all right because it is healthy. It is not healthy to add oil to your diet. If you are going to put any oil on, olive oil is better than other oils.

Reading about good fats and bad fats can be confusing. I will simplify the facts for you. Fats that are a natural part of natural wholesome foods are good for you. Fats that are added in processing or preparing foods are bad for you. If you still want to add fats to your food in processing, use monounsaturated fats such as extra-virgin olive oil. Fats are important to have in your diet, and the good fats appear in fish, nuts, seeds, avocado, and olives. The bad fats are the saturated fats, trans fats (hydrogenated and partially hydrogenated fats), and polyunsaturated fats. These fats are derived from processed foods or oils used to prepare foods. Avoid processed foods and added oils, and you will automatically avoid the bad fats.

I don't like to make specific fat gram recommendations because the numbers vary depending on your personal needs and goals. You could start simply removing all fat that is added in the cooking process. Also eliminate any added fats, such as cheese, cream, mayonnaise, and oily sauces used to dress the food. If you need a fat intake guideline, I would recommend you limit your fat intake to no more than 20-30 grams per day—perhaps up to 60 grams per day, depending on your height or whether you are weight balanced and active.

Water

Increase the amount of water in your diet because it is good for you. Most of your fluids should come in the form of natural and pure water. Drinking more water with your meals will also help fill your stomach to feel full faster, thereby helping you to achieve your weight loss goals. You should always keep yourself well hydrated to help your body flush toxins and wastes from your system.

Basic Meal Selection

As you can see, the types of food you select to eat can help you lose weight. High protein foods, fiber, and fluids will help satisfy your desire to eat in a healthy manner. They are good for you and reduce your hunger. Fat will also satisfy your hunger and is acceptable when it is a natural part of your protein food, such as the fat in meat.

You should also concentrate on eating natural, unaltered foods. Foods prepared with artificial preservatives, artificial colors, and flavorings include chemicals that can function as toxins in your body. Your body is not genetically developed to process and eliminate these artificial substances. Your body has a liver and kidneys to eliminate the naturally toxic byproducts of digestion but they are not programmed to eliminate unnatural foods. Your body may have difficulty processing these chemicals and eradicating them from your body. They will gradually damage your organs, tissues and cells decreasing your future longevity and functionality.

Your basic meals should be constructed carefully. Give higher priority to protein followed by fiber followed by carbohydrates. Here's what a basic meal should look like:

- Primary item to select is a lean meat for protein. The meal should start with the primary selection of protein rich meat source. The protein is healthy and will satisfy your hunger. Lean meats include poultry and fish. Lean red meats (tenderloin, low-fat ground meat) are good but less preferable. Meats should be prepared without added oils or sauces. The natural fat in lean meat is acceptable.
- Secondary item to select is a fiber source such as vegetables, beans, or legumes. These foods have high fiber content to fill you up. Like meats, they should be prepared without added oils or sauces. Meats and high-fiber foods should form the bulk of your meals.
- Tertiary item to select is a limited amount of carbohydrates as needed to fuel your body. Include a reasonable portion of bread, pasta, or rice, always choosing whole grains if possible. Carbohydrates should be eaten in amounts significantly less than you usually eat and will require the most adjustment, depending upon your level of obesity and your activity levels.

Your meals are built in this specific order of priority. Similarly, your weight loss plan should eliminate foods in the reverse order. The first foods you should begin eliminating or reducing are the carbohydrate fillers. Initially, cut the carbohydrate volume in half. If you are not losing weight, eliminate carbohydrates altogether.

If you are eating meals prepared in or with added oils and sauces and are not losing weight, you need to eliminate the oils and fats. If you are eating high sugar sweets and desserts and you are not losing weight, you need to eliminate sugars.

I will suggest some techniques to help you feel full from your meal.

- Combine different items to feel full. If you eat two pieces of bread and then eat a skinless, boneless chicken breast, you will not feel as full as if you had put the chicken breast in the bread as a sandwich. As another example, if you were to eat a chicken breast and some vegetables, cut the meat and vegetables into pieces and mix them. The more the foods are mixed together, the more you will fill your hunger. Mixing the foods makes the digestion process more complex. Your body has to work harder to digest the foods, and you will have a deeper sense of satiety because your stomach will feel fuller.

- To help you feel a sense of fullness, always focus on eating predominantly lean meats and protein. These foods will make you feel satisfied soon after the meal, and the feeling of fullness will continue for several hours.
- Drink a lot of water with your meal. The extra water will fill your stomach and help simulate the sensation of fullness and satiety.
- Increase the amount of fiber in the meal to help create fullness as well. Eating fiber will make you feel satisfied soon after the meal, and the feeling will continue for several hours as well.

After you have achieved a healthy weight, you can resume a healthy, balanced way of living. It is simply not possible to eat a balanced diet while you are fat, because eating a balanced diet then would only maintain your fat level. Although I advocate health and balance, you have to have some imbalance during the weight-loss period. It was your imbalance that led to obesity, so it will require imbalance in the opposite direction to lose the weight.

Label Criteria

The best way to read labels is to determine whether the foods are of a healthy composition. Use the Protein Fat Ratio and the Carbohydrate Fiber Ratio to help you select healthy meals. This is a simple tool to analyze and select meals. It is easy because you don't have to add up grams and calories during the day.

If you prefer to have specific calculations, then you can use the following criteria to help you read labels to select healthy foods. The following information includes ranges, and you can decide how aggressive to be. These numbers are also dependent upon your height, current weight, and activity level.

- Aim to increase your protein intake to 60-120 grams (depending upon your size and activity level).
- Add up fiber grams for a total of 25-30 grams eaten per day. This level should come from whole grain foods, beans, and vegetables. High fiber foods include vegetables, fruits, whole grain foods, leaf salad, beans, peas, lentils, and other legumes.
- The amount of carbohydrates (such as breads, pasta, rice and potatoes) and fruits you should be eating is much harder to specify and is dependent upon your activity level. As a starting point, I suggest cut-

ting your simple carbohydrate intake in half, not by counting, but by eating half the portion that you would typically eat. Over time, you can adjust your carbohydrate intake as needed based upon the results you are achieving.

- Aim to limit your fat intake to less than 20-30 grams (depending upon your size and activity level, perhaps up to 60 grams in select cases).

Chapter 8

Exercise in the Middle Way

You should have a balanced approach to your exercise regimen. Too little exercise, and you will not gain any benefit. Too much exercise can cause injury to your body. You have to find the right balance for yourself in terms of the frequency, duration, and degree of your exercise.

Exercise should be a supplement to your diet. The diet, plus your focus on how and what you eat, should be the primary basis for weight loss. The exercise is the secondary focus, but critical to losing weight. This approach will help you to realize that you can control your intake of food. Otherwise, you may fall into a routine of exercising to be able to eat. On occasion, this approach can be reasonable, but it will fail you if exercising-to-eat becomes chronic.

You have probably seen people exercising vigorously and regularly, yet you notice that those people remain overweight. They stay fat because they are exercising as a primary focus and as a way to justify overeating—perhaps going to an "all you can eat" brunch after the workout. These people are exercising excessively to be able to eat excessively. This system of exercising to eat might work after you become thin. Even then, it is not advisable because you risk falling into the trap of over-exercising and risking injury.

The primary goal of exercising is to be healthy. Therefore, the primary goal *during* exercise should be to avoid injury. Even after you become experienced, injury can always occur. Extreme exercise can lead to injury that will prevent you from exercising as you should. If you find yourself being injured repeatedly by your exercise, you may be exercising to extremes. If you keep a balanced approach, you can reduce injury frequency.

The Scale is Your Report Card

Use scales to monitor your weight loss progress. You should weigh the same or less each morning. You should weigh yourself at the same time every day in the same state of hydration, preferably first thing in the morning before eating or drinking anything. Hydration levels can easily change your weight reading. If you weigh yourself at night and compare it to the morning's weight, your reading will often be 1-2 pounds different by the morning, just because of dehydration.

The scale is the report card on how you are doing and gives you immediate feedback on the effectiveness of your efforts. If the scale isn't going down, you need to increase your efforts and cut back on food intake and/or increase exercise—or both.

Do not expect to see immediate results on a daily basis. The response on the scale will lag behind your weight-loss efforts. Use a body fat scale as another type of guide to your success. While losing weight, you should aim to see both your body weight and your body fat percentage decrease. After you have lost the appropriate weight, you can use the scale to monitor how well you maintain your weight and your body fat percentage.

You probably took a long time to put on added weight, and you will take some time to remove the weight. You may have put on one or two pounds per year. After twenty years, you'll have added twenty to forty extra pounds, much of it fat. You won't take 20 years to lose the added weight, but you should have a reasonable expectation of how fast you will lose it. You could go slowly and lose one pound a month with mild adjustment to your nutrition and activity levels. A more modest approach could be one or two pounds lost each week, and that amount of loss would require a more concentrated effort on reducing intake and increasing activity. You could start slowly, and as you develop confidence and change your perspective, you could gradually become more aggressive in your program.

As you start your exercise regimen, please plan the exercise into your daily schedule. Weight loss and exercise must be a top priority. You should be able to exercise at least three times a week for an hour at a time. You need to take care of yourself before you can take care of the others in your life. Make the commitment to yourself as a gift to your family. The time sacrifice in the short term will be more than made up by the long-term benefits of living longer and healthier.

Exercise Improves Your Quality of Life

The main goal of weight loss and exercise should be to lengthen the period of your healthy longevity. You know that a balanced, healthy way of living will benefit the quality of your life tomorrow as much as it extends your life. Healthy life choices today can improve the quality of your life as soon as tomorrow. By living well today, you will sleep well tonight. You will have sufficient energy to appreciate and enjoy life that day. Live your life with the intention to live forever. Live your life to improve the chance of a healthy and satisfying senior life.

The methods you use for exercise and the amount of exercise you do should also be balanced. There is a middle level that makes reasonable sense. Regular exercise is an important part of losing weight and of maintaining a healthy and functioning body. Exercise will also benefit your mind. Here is a list of some of the benefits of regular exercise:

- Improved mood and energy levels
- Antidepressant effect
- Stress and tension relief
- Cognitive improvement
- Improved immunity and decreased incidence of illness such as colds and flu.
- Improved sleep habits
- Improved mental and physical strength and stamina
- Appetite suppression and control
- Improved digestion and bowel function

Now you start to see the reality of a healthy life with exercise. Not exercising will cause you more difficulty and pain than the exercise itself. The physical and emotionally damaging effects of inactivity are far outweighed by the benefits of simply exercising. When you become active, you will feel mentally alert, emotionally stable, and physically strong so that you can get the most from your days and years. Exercise will improve your mind and, in turn, your stronger mind will help you exercise regularly. A positive cycle will form, and many important aspects of your life will improve.

Make it a Priority in Your Schedule

In the beginning, you may find it challenging to motivate yourself to get started. I hope you will realize that this challenge does not continue forever. Beginning each period of exercise will not always be a struggle. As you gain momentum and as exercise becomes a natural part of your routine, it will become automatic, a natural part of your day. You will no longer debate whether you should or shouldn't bother to exercise. Not exercising will become harder for you than exercising.

Having begun a program of exercise, you are likely to realize how poorly your body and mind feel and function on those days that you are unable to exercise as planned. You will naturally exercise regularly, happily, and painlessly. If and when you do feel any difficulty getting motivated, it should help you to know that only the beginning of your exercise session will be challenging. After you get started, your body will wake up. The first five or ten minutes will occasionally seem a little difficult, but soon you will fall into the rhythm and will feel good.

To begin, simply make the exercise schedule, and plan what you will be doing. Do it automatically. You get up every day and go to work because you have to. Seeing no options, you return every Monday morning. If you shift your perspective just a little and realize that exercise is similar in that you have no option, you will exercise without fighting yourself about it.

Learn to Make Exercise Part of Your Life

Start out slow and easy. Don't push yourself beyond the point where you feel like stopping. If you really feel like stopping, just stop. It is not necessary to make yourself suffer. The goal of the exercise is to improve your life. The most important step to accomplish in the first weeks is for you to learn how to make exercise fit easily into your schedule.

Over time, you may naturally find yourself increasing the intensity of exercise. Gradually, you may push yourself to do a little bit more. The positive effects of exercise on your life may leave you wanting more. You can slowly increase the amount and intensity of the exercise to an appropriate, safe level. Maintain conscious awareness, and find the right balance of frequency and intensity. You can tweak the frequency and intensity to increase your weight loss if you find that you are not making satisfactory progress. If you are not losing weight despite being at a high frequency and intensity of exercise, perhaps you need to focus attention on your diet. You may be exercising adequately but still eating inappropriately.

As you become more advanced, you may risk exercising too much. Let your body signal to you where to find the right balance. You should aim to feel a little sore for one or two days after the activity. If you do not feel any soreness, you may need to increase the intensity of your activity. If you feel extremely sore for more than two days, you are exercising too hard and should cut back the duration or the intensity level.

If you find yourself getting injured repeatedly, you should consider the adequacy of your warm-ups. Also consider that you may be exercising too frequently or intensely. Make sure that you are not restricting yourself to one particular type of activity that may make you likely to suffer an overuse injury.

Don't limit your exercise to one activity. Focusing too much on just one kind of exercise can increase the risk of acute injury, which would limit your ability to enjoy physical activity for the rest of your life.

Cross-training is essential. Mix up the activities you do as exercise. Cross-training will spread the physical stress to different parts of your body, reducing the chance of acute and chronic injury to any one part. Furthermore, you can have other parts of your body benefit from exercise. Limiting your exercise to running, for example, will not improve the health of your back and upper body.

It is a good idea to have a basic weekly routine that is varied with different types of exercise to condition all the muscles of your body. Sometimes you can substitute or add various activities to keep exercise interesting and fun. If on Sunday you typically run, on occasion you might substitute a trail and rock-climbing excursion. If on Thursday you typically swim, you might substitute paddling a canoe so you can enjoy the mental satisfaction of being outdoors. Mix it up and be active.

The details of how to exercise and how to create your exercise program are not the goal here. Every individual will have to create a program that suits their personality and way of living. No single plan or set of exercises can work for everyone.

Be mindful of what you learn as you create your individualized program. Develop a varied program that addresses all the parts of your body including legs, core, and upper body. Give yourself the benefits of aerobic conditioning and muscle strengthening. Mix some running, biking, swimming, and weight/resistance training into your routine. Many exercise options and combinations are possible to suit your personal circumstances.

- Morning: It is hard to adapt to at first but it can be done. Going for a run near your home or exercising in your home are good options. You can take a change of clothes with you to the gym and change into your work clothes afterward to go to your place of work.
- Lunch break: I don't recommend working out after lunch or instead of eating lunch because I advocate a peaceful break in the middle of your work day to have a relaxed lunch. I recommend having a meditative nap after lunch to help energize you for the rest of the day. However, if exercising during lunch is the only option, do it.
- After work or school: Preparing your gym bag the night before can make it easy for you to exercise before you go home. Exercising before dinner can help relieve your desire to eat after work, and the exercise will help relieve stress and can help curb your appetite for the remainder of the evening.
- After you get home in the evening: I do not recommend this schedule because after you get home, you often encounter many distractions that will make beginning your exercise program a challenge. Even if you are not distracted by other people, you can be tempted to grab a snack to eat while you relax after work. If you need to go home after work, try to exercise immediately after you get home. The longer you wait, the harder it will be to start exercising. Another option is to go back outside to exercise as late as eight or nine o'clock in the evening after you attend to the at-home responsibilities.
- Weekends: These days are excellent for exercise because you have all of a day to fit exercise into. I recommend exercising in the morning so you can enjoy the feeling of energy afterward. Exercising early also avoids any distractions that may arise during the day even on weekends. Regular exercising on weekends helps you curb your appetite so you can avoid overeating when you encounter a tempting weekend meal.
- Free moments: If you find that your evenings are busy with your children's activities, make the most of the opportunity to spend time with them and fit in your own exercise at the same time. If you take the children to a sports practice, bring your running shoes and run around the field.
- Your children are not an excuse to avoid exercise. They are a reason to exercise. Involve them in your workouts. Go for a run, and let your children ride their bikes. Do physical activities with your children.

Get them and yourself out of the house and be active. The children will benefit just as you do from physical exercise. They need physical activity to improve their physical and mental functioning. You can involve yourself in many activities with them, such as tennis, basketball, hiking, biking, rollerblading, ice skating, skiing, and even dancing. Enjoy the time with your children, for you will bond with them and become healthy together.

- Physical limitations are not excuses for not exercising. Do what you can and make the most of your capacity rather than using it as an excuse. So don't whine and cry that your knees bother you. When your knees hurt, go swimming. If your shoulder hurts, run. When running hurts, ride a bike. Remember: you are benefiting your mind and your body when you exercise.

- You can choose from many activities for exercise. A few of the activities may form your basic schedule, but I highly recommend incorporating variation on occasion in addition or as a substitute for the basic schedule. The obvious types of exercise are the gym exercises. They are very effective and provide different exercises to address all the parts of your body, both aerobic and muscle resistance. The gym is a good place to start, and it can form the basis of your exercise regimen. From there, you can branch out to other locations with a greater variety of activities.

- Walking casually for twenty minutes three times a week is acceptable, but that approach is probably not adequate for you to achieve significant weight loss. This much exercise is certainly better than nothing. However, don't fool yourself into thinking that minimal exercise will produce a loss of forty to fifty pounds within a reasonable amount of time. Yet if walking casually for only twenty minutes is the most that you can do because of your mental or physical capacity, do that much.

Walking can be more beneficial if performed vigorously for a lengthy period. In any physical activity, the more intensely you exercise, the shorter period of time required. If your exercise is less vigorous, you will have to increase the duration of the workout to achieve the same benefits. Walking at a fast pace on an incline treadmill for thirty to sixty minutes will have significantly more benefits than walking for the same period on a flat surface. Walking is also minimally abusive to your knees and will help them to last much longer than excessive running will. Outdoor walking with speed and vigor on hills and stairs is also excellent.

- I do recommend running as an excellent form of exercise, but it has to be done in a reasonable, balanced manner. Running can be an important part of your regimen but should not be the primary focus. It is best not to do only one form of exercise, and running for an hour several times each week is likely to compromise the long-term health of your knees. You should find a reasonable balance and accept the risks of your decisions.

  If you choose to run, be cautious about your technique. It is crucial that you run so that you reduce the pounding on your joints. It is better to run softly, lightly and slowly. Run so that your heel touches first and rolls smoothly forward to the toes. Your foot should not land flat on the surface because doing so will strain your knees and hip joints. Always exercise with the intention to use the muscles, not to strain the ligaments or stress the joints. Outdoor running is efficient because you don't have to drive to the gym or use special equipment other that good running shoes. Anyone can run because the activity doesn't require athletic talent.

- Riding a bike is a safe way to exercise your lower body and get aerobic benefits. It is highly recommended because of the low stress load on your joints. You can ride the stationary bike at the gym when the weather is bad. Outdoor biking is also a good way to enjoy being outdoors and get satisfying exercise at the same time.

The exercise options available to you are nearly endless. Find what you prefer and do it. You can choose tennis, basketball, soccer, hiking, canoeing or kayaking, rollerblading, ice skating, dancing, and skiing. And then you can start a list of your own!

Aerobic exercise is important, but weight resistance training should also be included in your program. Weight resistance training can improve your overall physical health in a way that aerobic exercise alone will not. Weight resistance will improve the strength of your skeletal structure, bones, muscles, and tendons. It can have significant impact on your weight loss program and can help with weight control as well.

Weight resistance training stimulates your muscle and thereby increasing your metabolism that last well beyond the training period. For the next few days as your muscles recover from the exercise, they will continue to burn calories. The muscle recovery process itself puts a high metabolic demand on your system and helps to burn calories and fat. Furthermore, increasing your muscle mass increases the number of calories your body can burn daily even without exercise. This is like increasing the size of your engine from four to eight cylinders, burning more fuel. So you see that you can increase your metabolism. Muscles burn the calories. The more muscle mass you have, the more effectively you will burn the calories you ingest.

Here are some ideas for incorporating weight resistance training into your workout schedule.

- Free weights and exercise machines are excellent for exercising a variety of muscles. The machines allow you to effectively target all the major muscle groups so that you can exercise your entire body.
- Always warm up before any activity. You increase the risk of injury if you begin immediately exercising at full speed and maximum intensity. As your body temperature rises and you start to sweat, you can increase the intensity or can transition to the more strenuous activity. Light running or biking is an excellent way to warm up for any activity. Starting out slowly and gradually will warm your muscles and increase the flexibility of your tendons and joints. Warming up is especially important for older people because, as the body ages, the tendons become stiffer and less pliable.
- Stretching is best done after the body has been warmed up. When the tendons are cold, stiff, and rigid, they are prone to stress, strain, tears, and rupture. After the body is warmed up, the tendons will be lubricated and ready for stretching.
- The tendons are also prone to injury during exercise. Never extend your joints beyond ninety degrees under excess tension. Range of motion exercise beyond ninety degrees is acceptable only if performed without excess tension. Keep all movements within the muscle action range, which is less than ninety degrees. When the joints are extending beyond that limit, the tendons will be stressed excessively and are at risk for straining or tearing. The tendons are like rubber bands in youth, but they turn into tightly woven ropes as you age. The only way to safely exercise your tendons is by stretching, them when they are warm, loose, and flexible.

Do something! Do anything! Move your body. Get busy. Stop sitting around. If the only thing you can do is walk, then walk. Allow yourself to make no excuses. Instead, make a conscious decision to get moving!

Chapter 9
Guideposts for Healthy Living

As you begin applying the middle way to your food and exercise program, having a list of reminders may be useful for you. I have collected a number of guideposts for getting started on your program. My hope is that these guideposts can help you plan what you eat and the ways you exercise to maintain your body as you follow the middle way.

Eat more protein.
>Increase the amount of lean meat portions in your meals and snacks. These portions should come from fish, poultry and lean red meats. High protein foods will make you feel fuller, faster and for longer. When you reach your weight-loss goal, you can increase the frequency of red meat portions.

Eat more fiber.
>Fiber is good for your colon and will help you feel fuller faster and longer. Substitute the simple carbohydrates with high fiber carbohydrates, such as high fiber vegetables. When you are slim, increase your intake of whole fruits.

Eat less simple carbohydrates.
>Simple carbohydrates may fill you up in the short term but will ultimately lead to your feeling hungrier sooner. Reduce the amount of white bread, pasta, potato, processed cereals, rice, sodas, and fruit juice in your meals. Do not add any sugar to your meals. Do not eat any sugary sweets, candies, or desserts. Fruits are good for you, but the number of portions should be controlled in order for you to lose

weight. When you become fit and remain active, you may reasonably increase fruit portions to fuel your body.

Eat less fat.
> Completely eliminate any oils and fats that are added to prepare or dress your meal. Do not include cheeses, mayonnaise, creams, cooking oils, butter, margarine, and sauces. Nuts are good for you but should be minimized if you wish to lose weight. When you are fit, be more flexible within reason in choosing nuts as part of your meals.

Drink more water.
> Water is good for your body, and if your drink more before and during your meals, you will feel fuller faster.

Increase your activity level.
> When your level of activity goes up, you will increase your metabolism. You can do some form of exercise to increase your metabolic rate. Aerobic exercise is good. Resistance training will enhance muscle metabolism.

Change your perspective of reality.
> Realize that eating healthy and exercising regularly can bring you more happiness than eating too much and not exercising.

Don't obsess about food.
> Learn to be happy without giving the type and amount of food too much value and importance in your life. Don't believe what you have been told by marketers. You can be happy without the objects and foods you believe will make you happy. Happiness is within your mind. Find joy and happiness in your life outside of food.

Create a peaceful environment.
> Limit your exposure to situations that tempt you to forget your middle way. Avoid situations that will tempt your desire to eat in an unhealthy manner. Take time for meditation and exercise, which will increase your sense of inner peace. Remember that you have control over your mind, so don't let it become filled with temptation and fear.

Eat only when you're really hungry.
> True hunger in your stomach should be your dinner bell, not your mind.

Eat only what you should.
> Think about how much you legitimately should eat before you start. Eat only that amount, realizing that you will feel full soon. Wait for that full feeling to develop up to 1 hour after eating.

Eat smaller meals more frequently.
> Plan to eat the right amount to satisfy your hunger and that will lead you to have legitimate feelings of hunger again in approximately 3-4 hours. Every 3 hours if eating 5 small meals a day. Up to every 4 hours if eating 4 meals per day. You should be getting hungry every few hours because you ate reasonably at the prior meal.

Eat similar foods at each meal.
> Consistency and lack of variability in types and size of meals will allow you to learn the appropriate amounts that will reasonably satisfy your hunger without overeating. This consistency in food choices will also allow you to make small adjustments to your diet according to the results you are achieving in weight loss.

Take smaller bites and slow down.
> This approach to dining can enhance your pleasure from food and simultaneously make you healthy.

Use a scale daily to monitor your progress.
> Weighing yourself gives you a report card on your efforts. If you are losing weight, keep up the good work. If you are not losing weight, be more aggressive in restricting food intake and increasing exercise. The scale doesn't lie. If you are exercising while dieting you will be losing pounds in the form of fat and not muscle. If dieting without exercise you will likely be losing fat and muscle. You could use a scale with body fat measuring to help you as well.

Read labels only for information.
> It is reasonable to read labels to monitor you diet. The Protein Fat Ratio and the Carbohydrate Fiber Ratio are simple easy ways to

select good meals. Do not get carried away adding calories as it is not possible to sustain a rigid formula of counting calories and preparing specific diet plan meals. Remember that the quantity of food you should take in depends on your height, current weight, and activity level. Aim to increase your protein intake to 60-120 grams. Aim to increase fiber to 25-30 grams. Aim to limit your fat intake to less than 20-30 grams.

Use the Protein Fat Ratio and the Carbohydrate Fiber Ratio to choose foods.
The Protein Fat Ratio is used to maximize protein intake with as little fat as possible. Therefore, the protein/fat ratio should be above 3 preferably and more than 2 at a minimum. You can calculate this ratio by taking the protein grams and dividing by the fat grams.

The Carbohydrate Fiber Ratio is used to minimize carbohydrate while maximizing fiber and therefore the carbohydrate/fiber ratio should be less than 10, in general. Calculate this by taking the carbohydrate grams and dividing by the fiber grams. Use these ratios to help you select healthy meals. It may be a little confusing to remember. To help, keep in mind that you want to <u>maximize</u> protein so the Protein Fat Ratio should be <u>over</u> 3. You want to <u>minimize</u> carbohydrates so the Carbohydrate Fiber Ratio should be <u>less</u> than 10.

Build your meals carefully.
Eat more proportionally of higher priority foods. To lose weight, eliminate progressively the items of lower priority to reach your weight goals. Use the Protein Fat Ratio and the Carbohydrate Fiber Ratio to confirm that your meals produce an objectively correct ratio in your diet. The priority progression shows you the order in which you are to choose foods. The guide indicates the importance of different food types in your diet. The guide also tells you how to increase or decrease food types according to their desired effect. For example, in order to lose weight, increase the foods nearer the top of the list, and decrease the foods nearer the bottom. To gain weight, decrease the foods nearer the top, and increase the foods nearer the bottom of the list.

- Proteins from lean meats such as fish, poultry, and lean cuts of red meat

- Fiber from vegetables, beans, and other legumes
- Carbohydrates from whole grains breads, cereals, and pastas
- Whole fruits
- Nuts
- Added oils and sauces
- Desserts and processed snack foods
- Sodas and fruit juices

References

Harvard School of Public Health, www.hsph.harvard.edu/nutritionsource

Natow, Annette B., Jo-Ann Heslin. 1997. *The Pocket Protein Counter.* Pocket Books. New York.

National Academy of Sciences, Institute of Medicine. Food and Nutrition Board. *Dietary Reference Intakes for Energy, Carbohydrate, Fiber, Fat, Fatty Acids, Cholesterol, Protein, and Amino Acids.* (2002/2005), www.iom.edu

United States Department of Agriculture, Agricultural Research Service, www.ars.usda.gov

About the Author

Emil Payman Moshedi, M.D., was born and raised in Maryland. He has a bachelors degree in Zoology from the George Washington University. He received his medical degree from the University of Maryland School of Medicine. He completed his internship in Internal Medicine at George Washington University. He was subsequently a scientist at the National Institutes of Health and received a National Research Service Award. His experience there led to the development of his patent on a medication for the prevention of heart attacks and strokes. He has also published numerous articles from his research in scientific journals. He then decided to do a residency in Ophthalmology and is board certified specializing in cataract, glaucoma, and diabetic eye surgery.

Although, Dr. Moshedi is a full time Eye Surgeon, he has always had a personal and academic interest in health and fitness. After years of study and stressful work he was physically overweight and emotionally drained. As an ophthalmologist he has an interest in how the brain visualizes the world and wondered how to see the reality of nutrition and fitness. He developed a philosophy for health and fitness that helped him transform his overweight body and unstable mind. Many of his colleagues had repeatedly asked him to share his experience with them and their patients. He has counseled both physicians and patients. As a trainer he takes the approach of training the mind as the primary focus rather than simply teaching exercise techniques. He has since written *The Middle Way Diet* to share his philosophy on nutrition and exercise.

978-0-595-41097-2
0-595-41097-9

Printed in the United States
95723LV00010B/2/A